ENLARGING THE THERAPEUTIC CIRCLE

The Therapist's Guide to Collaborative Therapy with Families and Schools

ENLARGING THE THERAPEUTIC CIRCLE

The Therapist's Guide to Collaborative Therapy with Families and Schools

Robert Sherman, Ed.D.
Adaia Shumsky, Ed.D.
Yvonne B. Rountree, Ph.D.

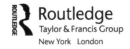
Routledge
Taylor & Francis Group
New York   London

First published by

BRUNNER/MAZEL, INC.
19 Union Square West
New York, New York 10003

This edition published 2012 by Routledge

Routledge	Routledge
Taylor & Francis Group	Taylor & Francis Group
711 Third Avenue	27 Church Road
New York, NY 10017	Hove East Sussex BN3 2FA

Library of Congress Cataloging-in-Publication Data

Sherman, Robert
    Enlarging the therapeutic circle: the therapist's guide to collabora-
tive therapy with families and schools / Robert Sherman, Adaia
Shumsky, Yvonne B. Rountree
        p.   cm.
    Includes bibliographical references and index
    ISBN 0-87630-739-X
    1. Child psychotherapy. 2. Ecopsychiatry. 3. Adolescent
psychotherapy. 4. Psychiatric consultation. I. Shumsky, Adaia.
II. Rountree, Yvonne. III. Title.
RJ505.E25S54 1994
618.92'8914—dc20   94-12393
                                                          CIP

We dedicate this book to family, friends, and colleagues who have given us their full support;

to those who have mentored us professionally and in life;

and to those who have labored to develop successful collaborative models that provided a useful foundation for our own work.

Contents

Foreword

Finally we have a book that addresses what research and common sense tell us: children who dysfunction do it as a result of the systems in which they reside. Although the data has been available, professionals have not been willing to broaden their therapeutic circles and theoretical frameworks in order to change their professional practices.

The exciting thing about *Enlarging the Therapeutic Circle* is that it will make a real impact. This book is not just words or more of the same. Real, permanent, second-order change can be produced by using the authors' ideas. Do you have the courage to read further? If so, you will need to abandon your usual, comfortably ineffective methods of helping.

The authors present a strong rationale for ecosystemic intervention and a realistic discussion of the types of school and family resistance. The authors have practiced this approach for over 25 years in a variety of settings and truly understand what they are presenting. Effective treatment for children and adolescents must include those persons with whom they interact the most and who are the most influential/powerful in their lives. Children and adolescents are firmly entrenched in their social system. They both act upon and are products of this world. What is acceptable or not is determined by the rules and the boundaries of the system. However, schools, families, and other haunts of children and adolescents do not always have clear or consistent rules. Rules also vary from system to system.

This book shows how to develop and apply consistent treatment plans through collaboration among children, families, and schools. The therapist functions as an initiator, coordinator, and consultant.

The ideas of the authors are based upon a sound theoretical framework, that of Adlerian psychology. This positive approach allows for holistic, developmental, and systemic formulations.

This is a bold book that has balanced vision with the practical details needed by the therapist to be truly effective. If I wore a hat, I would take it off as a sign of great respect for these authors and their ideas.

The weakness of this book is the weakness of all books—that no matter how good the words are, readers tend to do what they learned or feel comfortable with, rather than what really works. This brings to mind the oft-quoted Sufi story of the man on his hands and knees under the streetlamp, crawling around searching for his lost watch. A passerby asks, "May I help you?" and gets down on his hands and knees looking under the streetlamp. The passerby asks, "Where did you lose your watch?" and the man says, "Over there in the dark stairwell." The passerby then asks the obvious question, "If you lost it over there, why are you looking out here?" "Because the light is better here," the man answers.

I challenge you, are you willing to enlarge your therapeutic circle and go under the stairs to join Sherman, Shumsky, and Rountree?

JON CARLSON, Psy.D., Ed.D., ABPP
Distinguished Professor, Governors
  State University
President, International Association of
  Marriage and Family Counselors

Preface

The authors are all psychologists currently affiliated with Queens College in New York. We have a long history of working with children and families, both directly in schools as school practitioners and collaboratively as private clinicians and university professors. Queens College has maintained collaborative relationships with schools for many purposes almost since its founding in 1937. The Counselor Education Program has initiated a total of 14 free open-door counseling services affiliated with public schools, religious institutions, Ys, and community agencies since 1968. Graduates of our Family Therapy Program have established school districtwide or individual school-based treatment and training programs affiliated with the College. Therefore we are involved in a long tradition of collaborative treatment and training. We thought that it would be worthwhile to share some of our experiences, and those of other like-minded colleagues, by preparing a guidebook for involving therapists, children, families, and school personnel in the joint adventure of bringing about constructive change, especially for children at risk.

This book is based on the thesis that therapists of all theoretical persuasions can often best help children and adolescents by including in their treatment those persons whom children interact with the most as well as those persons who hold the most influence. Television programmers possibly best meet these criteria because of the amount of time children spend in front of the TV screen, but they are neither available nor necessarily therapeutic. The family and the school usually can be. Further, both the family and the school are the two institutions specifically designated by society to socialize and guide children in their growth and development. It is also these institutions, as well as the police/court system, that are most likely to define a child as being in difficulty and in need of therapeutic help.

Children and adolescents are firmly embedded in social systems. The systems define the meaning and value of their behavior and give them an identity through the evaluations and the assignment of roles. In turn, children, through their behavior and the roles that they assume, profoundly influence the systems of which they are a part. When a parent labels a child as "bad" or a teacher labels him as a "failure," the child is not only receiving an evaluation of his behavior, he is being given an identity in the group. By assuming a label, the child further begins to act out the role implied by the label, thus impacting on the group.*

What constitutes "bad" or "failure" are meanings assigned within the specific group. When the child does not conform to the expectations of the system, he gets into trouble with other members, particularly the power structure. This is true in family, school, church, community, or peer group. In each of these groups the child is part of the larger whole and, therefore, he is expected to behave according to the rules of each system.

System rules are not always clear or consistent. Nor are the rules necessarily similar from one system or set of circumstances to another. In the classroom children may be expected to raise their hand and get permission in order to speak, while at home they may have to interrupt others to get a word in. Following the rules can therefore be quite confusing. For a rule to stick the members must cooperate in observing it. Rejection of a rule by one or more members is really the subject of interpersonal conflict and rebellion against authority. Children, who are rarely consulted in the formulation of rules, may sometimes find reason to challenge them. This is equally true for "therapeutic" plans created for the child in trouble by parents, schools, or courts. Children also try to make and enforce rules with others in their lives and often find that the others refuse to comply. The children then feel treated unjustly, unlovingly, or demeaningly, concluding that they are victims.

---

* The reader will notice that for the sake of editorial convenience therapists are frequently referred to as she and clients as he and great care has been taken to use nonsexist language.

A child at risk is one who meets one of three criteria: his physical health is endangered, such as by disease, physical abuse, or substance abuse; his feelings about himself and the world are negative and discouraging; or his interactions with other people are ineffective or disapproved of by others. This third criterion applies as well to the adolescent who does not conform to the rules of his antisocial gang.

If a child's behavior is disturbing to adults, the adults take action to forge a greater conformity through discussion, instruction, disciplinary action, medical treatment, mental health treatment, legal proceedings, or some form of banishment. When adults are disturbed by what the child is doing or experiencing it is typical that they will initiate treatment with the child as the identified client who has something wrong with him.

The therapist typically undertakes the treatment of this child as the referred identified patient as if the problem were somehow all within the child. The therapist is instructed and usually paid by the dissatisfied adults. The adults' presenting problem might be that the child needs help to behave properly: he's too shy, too passive, too hostile, too uncooperative, too fat, or too sad. The child's presenting problem might be one or all of the following: my parents or teachers are unfair and pick on me all the time and never listen to what I have to say; I can't or don't want to do what they want me to do; or I'm not good enough, smart enough, accepted enough, loved enough.

Because the behavior arises, takes place, and is evaluated in a social context, it is more efficient to enlist the assistance of other participants in the system to bring about constructive change within that social system.

The school has the advantage of a professional staff, including mental health personnel, who could participate knowledgeably in a treatment plan applied consistently in the therapy office, school, and home. Developing and applying a consistent treatment plan is possible if it is prepared in collaboration with the child, family, and school. The therapist is here seen as the initiator, consultant, and coordinator for these activities.

By working collaboratively with both the school and the family, the therapist can greatly increase her power and therapeutic options. It also puts her in a position to win the trust and confidence of those who can refer many more clients to her private or agency practice. This book describes the rationale and methodology for building a collaborative practice with families and schools, including the possibility of consultant contract practices, which can also be applied to working with other institutions.

The authors think holistically, developmentally, and systemically about human behavior. We believe that continuing patterns of behavior are purposive and instrumental in attaining particular goals. The goals are in the service of individual and systemic beliefs and myths or to fulfill the rules of the ongoing interactional pattern among the members of the group that maintain the group as it is. If a child continues to act or "misbehave" in the same way, probably others in the family or school are eliciting or reinforcing that behavior by their reciprocal actions in a complementary pattern. Often, the very efforts to bring about change reinforce the status quo. For example, a parent criticizes her son for not doing a chore. The child feels put down and picked upon and therefore feels justified in avoiding doing that chore and others. This upsets the parent who criticizes and nags the son, who then feels even greater need to resist or to get revenge.

The authors further believe that a human organization is created and constantly recreated by the ongoing dynamic inputs of its individual members interacting among themselves. However, the organization also greatly influences the behavior of each of its members through its structure, demands, and myths. Therefore, we need to study and work with both the individual and the organization.

Children at risk are primarily identified by school personnel, family members, the police/court system, and sometimes by themselves. We observe that sometimes a presenting problem in one system really is a function of a problem in another system. For example, the acting-out student may be fighting to establish or maintain his individuality or sense of personhood in an enmeshed family; or he may be trying to lure attention away from upsetting and threatening parental fighting.

Based on the above and related beliefs, the authors advocate that it is useful and effective to study and treat children intrapsychically and sytemically in the context of their lives developmentally, culturally, and within the important systems of which they are members.

The first chapter of the book presents the history and theoretical rationale for therapists to work collaboratively with families and schools. The advantages, issues, obstacles, and directions are discussed. There are many issues and concerns that generally arise in such collaboration. Among them are who will be responsible for what, especially in overlapping areas of concern? How best to manage different professional ethical and legal codes as they influence the work? Who will keep what kinds of records? What information will be shared with whom and under what circumstances? What problems arise around issues of confidentiality? How are differing individual, family, professional, school, agency, and practice missions, cultures, values, and languages to be managed? Methods for utilizing the family and the school as support systems are also covered.

To help the therapist consult more effectively, descriptive concepts about how the school and family are organized as systems and how to utilize those systems for treatment are elaborated in Chapter 2. Information useful to therapists includes how schools generally organize their mental health services, what personnel and resources are available, the kinds of test results and records utilized, as well as special laws and programs.

Chapter 3 provides reports of five different successful models for therapist/family/school collabration initiated by individual therapists and agencies and what they have in common as well as the differences among them. Each model is discussed in terms of its theory and rationale, process or steps, and hoped for outcomes.

Schools and universities have been active in developing school-based family therapy clinics. Six school-based models are presented in Chapter 4, including one functioning in Japan. Again, each model is discussed in terms of its theory and rationale, process or steps, and outcomes. The commonalities and differences among them are identified.

Chapters 5 through 7 deal with the nuts and bolts of collaboration from the initial identification and referral processes through assessment, feedback, treatment, and follow-up. Resources and procedures are elaborated for such purposes as identifying children and adolescents at risk and bringing them into therapy. Some of the issues discussed are attitudes toward therapy, finances, mobility, making and obtaining referrals, outreach efforts, including local agencies, and maintaining the children in therapy. Methods and guidelines for doing collaborative assessment per se are the subjects of Chapter 6. Chapter 7 deals specifically with methods and guidelines for collaborative treatment and follow-up procedures.

The reader can therefore draw from a wide range of strategies that work.

In order to demonstrate that collaborations as advocated in this book can be practical and effective, Chapters 8 and 9 relate two detailed case studies involving many participating persons and institutions. The case in Chapter 8 revolves around several siblings who are children very much at risk. The case is initiated by a therapist in private practice who also coordinates the case. The presentation is largely clinically oriented within a collaborative framework. Chapter 9 concerns a poor, multiproblem, single-parent, recent immigrant family with an 8-year-old boy at risk. The case is more school- and agency-based. The collaborative process itself is emphasized in detail with some clinical material included.

Chapter 10 presents a view into the future. It examines changes and trends that either facilitate or inhibit collaboration in our society and in our professions. It also portrays some ideas about the therapist of the future.

This book, then, provides the therapist with both the theoretical concepts and practical models and methods for expanding her or his practice into collaborative work with families and schools and other local agencies. In the process of doing so, the skilled therapist may well expect to provide more effective services, become better known and respected in the community, and increase her or his private or agency referral base. This latter outcome is particularly important in view of the changes taking place nationally and locally in the ways in which services are to be provided under the influence and competition of managed care programs.

Although the book is written largely from the perspective of the clinician working in private practice or in an agency, it is also a particularly useful guide to school support service personnel and administrators, both in working with outside agencies and therapists and in setting up a school-based clinic. Students in any mental health training program will achieve a broader perspective of how they can work collaboratively in an interdisciplinary framework. They will learn the specifics of how and why to do so.

The models presented herein can readily be adapted to working with such other systems as hospitals, agencies, the criminal justice system, businesses, and managed care operations.

Acknowledgments

The authors wish to thank several people who were generous in sharing written materials or information on projects in which they were involved. Among them are Pearl Dorsey, June Oats, Barry Schwarcz, Howard Weiss, and Patricia Woods. Special thanks are due to Dr. Professor Kayoko Murace of Taishi University and Professor Eiji Koizumi of Waseda University in Tokyo, Japan, for granting us personal interviews and sharing with us their unique insights concerning school and family relationships in Japan. Their work offers a broad, multicultural perspective that we have attempted to maintain in our exploration of the issue of helping children at risk.

We are grateful to Julia C. Green, who provided the case study for and ably coauthored Chapter 8. Beverly Weinstein helped us to identify appropriate case studies and connected us with Julia.

Mark Tracten, our publisher, and Natalie Gilman, our editor, assisted us in refining the concept and direction of this book in ways that we believe greatly enhanced it. Of course, the authors accept sole responsibility for the contents of this book. Our thanks also go to Patricia Wolf, our managing editor, who capably saw to the actual production of the book.

CHAPTER 1

=========

WHY ENLARGE THE THERAPEUTIC CIRCLE?

I. INTRODUCTION: THE WORLD OF THE CHILD

There are many advantages for the therapist and child under his or her care to expand on the world inside the child's head and to go beyond to the total context in which the child lives and interacts.

Obviously, children inhabit many worlds: home, extended family, streets, playgrounds, school, community, and religious institutions. They are imbued with the culture and ethnicity of the family, neighborhood, and larger society. They are immersed in what adults and peers around them are doing. They are exposed to mass media. They do relatively little that is not learned from others and reinforced by the demands and reciprocal behavior of others. Their very identity is shaped by the evaluations and labels put on them by other people and the roles they assume in the various organizations in which they participate, either by choice, social convention, or social pressure. The children often find themselves under the disparate pressures of moving toward both conformity within their many cultures and rebelling against them to establish some form of individual identity and existence in a larger culture that stresses ego and individuality.

1

Children must somehow adapt to all the diverse cultures of the family, street, church, school, and larger society through which they move. There are relatively few homogeneous neighborhoods in our urban communities. For example, there are well over 100 distinct ethnic groups living in the Queens borough of New York City. Culture specifies how one is to give meaning to and cope with the challenges and stages of life. Both opportunities and constraints in behavior are prescribed—thou shalt and thou shalt not. Each culture is a rich lodestone of myths about life and the world: us and them.

Adler (in Ansbacher & Ansbacher, 1956) proposed long ago that the individual is socially embedded but that he or she approaches each situation and relationship in terms of a unified life-style developed in childhood. Gergen (1991) asserts that in such a diverse society as ours, which lacks homogeneous rules, structures, and definitions of reality, the person is bombarded with inconsistent information and demands and varying concepts of right and wrong, good and true. Gergen claims that the self becomes saturated and diffuse, creating dilemmas of identity. He believes that the person in fact constructs a different personal and systemic reality depending on his or her relationship to each individual, situation, and institution.

Add to the cultural mix the stresses of poverty, drugs, violence, divorce, remarriage, teen births, physical, sexual, and emotional abuse, as well as other social and health disadvantages. These beset so many of our youngsters, especially in the urban environment.

It is not surprising that many families and many neighborhoods appear to function in very chaotic and often oppositional ways. Interestingly, Hawkins (1993) describes such families as "random families," which "at their best...are creative, vibrant, joyfully disjointed..." (p. 60). The trick, he says, is to turn chaos into creativity by helping them to find lost significant information in the overload of information they receive; pass that information along; make connections with people by staying long enough in the same place; reduce the number of solutions from which to choose; and reduce the number of people involved. He suggests that these types of

creative persons are individualistic and have difficulty working cooperatively or in teams.

We find, therefore, that we are dealing with a very complex and confusing set of ingredients that make up the world
of children and families, especially those at risk or in therapy.

As the major formal socializing agencies, the home and
the school hold the primary responsibility for helping the
child make sense of all this complexity and pursue a constructive developmental path through life. Typically, when
something is amiss, it is most likely reflected in the behavior
within the family and the school. When therapists are called
in to assist, it is helpful to pool their resources and work together with the family and the school in a unified way to help
the child through the maze. If each of these institutions is
pulling and pushing in different directions to "help" the child,
the problem may be reinforced rather than alleviated as the
child is further "saturated."

The cultural traditions of many families are such that they
are unlikely to seek help from a psychotherapist or to believe
in psychotherapy. For such families there are only two points
of entry into psychotherapy: a mandate from the courts or
from the school. Thus, for many children at risk, it is only
through the school that the therapist will even become involved.

II. ADVANTAGES FOR THE THERAPIST OF
WORKING WITH FAMILIES AND SCHOOLS

A. Development of Theory and Techniques

The rapid development of family therapy theories and
methods makes available to all mental health practitioners a
body of knowledge and skills for approaching and working
effectively with the family. Most schools of psychotherapy have
now evolved family therapy procedures consonant with their
own theories. Therefore any mental health practitioner is
likely to find a handy family therapy model within her own
theoretical orientation. Some basic general principles are

described in Chapter 2 to point the direction for practical collaborative family work.

By engaging the family and school, the therapist adds enormously to the therapeutic options and treatment plans available. For example, emotional and practical supports can be created to encourage the child, such as tutoring, different school placements, and changes in child-rearing practices. Family problems affecting the child can be uncovered and attended to. School records, family medical records, and family history may be utilized for diagnosis. The child may be given individualized school assignments or be involved in new school activities.

The therapist has available a host of special structured techniques that can be adapted to her theoretical model and that can be brought into play. For example, The Family Meeting, Nondemand Communication, and the Negotiating Guide (Sherman, Oresky, & Rountree, 1991) and Early Recollections, Creating Analogous Situations, Caring Days, Strategic Alliances, The Winner's Bet, and creating the Surrogate Family Group (Sherman & Fredman, 1986) can be very useful. Similarly, reframing, stories, experiments, and positive blame are techniques that can be used in school and with parents (Kral in de Shazer & Kral, 1986).

Schaeffer (1988) presents a wide range of techniques, such as photo therapy, videotherapy, animal therapy, and the creation of life books. Nelson and Trepper (1993) gathered 101 techniques, many of which are very helpful tools for working with the family. Albert (1989) describes many techniques and provides a model that can be used in the classroom. Standardized tests are or can be administered by the school. There are a multitude of parent education and marriage enrichment programs commercially available. These are but a few of the many techniques and models described in the literature that add to the therapist's power and skills when she works with family and school as well as with the individual client.

It is also possible to formulate a treatment plan that may include some ways of impacting on the child's peer group in school on behalf of the child or through the child. Other children may be encourgaged to behave differently toward the particular child at risk, or the child already in therapy may be encouraged to take on a constructive leadership role among other children who are at risk. Such a plan may induce a powerful spread of effect.

B. The Family

Many institutions and neighborhood peers influence the child or youth. But the most enduring and impactful relationships more typically are those involved in the family. The family has a deep vested interest in its members. It is in the family that the children's primary needs are likely to be met or unmet and their health and development fostered or frustrated. There is a legacy of history, loyalty, needs, and goals that bind family members together in caring, albeit sometimes angry or hurtful, ways. Many of the children's strengths that can be utilized for treatment purposes are derived from their position in the family and family values. Similarly, many problems exhibited by the children are rooted in the family system. For example, children who are repeatedly criticized in order to improve performance may well come to believe that they can never be good enough as human beings or successful in life.

The family, because of its more limited size, mission, and caring, usually is an environment more interested in and available to therapeutic influence than most other larger, even more complex systems in the children's world.

C. The School

Although school truancy is a problem that may bring many children and youths at risk to the attention of family and authorities, the vast majority of children spend 6 to 7 hours each day for 180 or more days per year in school. And movements are now afoot to extend the school year. Next to the family, the school probably has the most enduring influence on most children, even those who are alienated in the school environment. Indeed, the authors observe that many students at risk are in fact alienated at school or hang out with antisocial or "drop-out" groups of youngsters alienated from the system.

The school is a structured environment designed to promote the learning, growth, and development of young people. It is staffed by trained professionals in teaching, administration, and support service personnel, such as psychologists, social workers, counselors, nurses, and other specialists, depending on the size and mission of the school. Few people or institutions attain the ideals to which they subscribe. Nevertheless, schools generally do provide a cadre of caring and interested professionals who work hard on behalf of the children under their care. This is also true of inner city schools across the nation often criticized as failures. Most school personnel are happy to work cooperatively with other experts to help their charges. Their knowledge of the children based on interacting with them for so many hours is invaluable. School resources such as testing programs, counseling services, extracurricular activities, special class placements, observational reports, and supervisory staff are examples of important assets to a therapist who knows how to reach out and connect with them to form creative partnerships.

It is also true that situations in school may promote or reinforce a child's difficulty, ranging from problems with peers to personality clashes with inept teachers to misplacement educationally to a war of competing wills. School interactions may severely discourage the student and lead to low self-esteem, withdrawal, or rebellious behavior. The criticism, evaluation, and labeling of children in school may also have severe negative consequences in the formulation of a person's identity as a failure, or not good enough, or stupid, or bad. Correcting such situations may well require the cooperation of school staff.

Because the school to a large degree is a professionally controlled environment, it too is both more susceptible to and open to practical therapeutic intervention than other systems in the child's world.

The therapist, standing outside the system and respected as an expert in her field, may be able to add valuable perceptions and effective suggestions as part of a treatment plan conjointly developed in a respectful, creative partnership with the school. Chapter 2 provides some general principles for working with the school as a system.

III. LARGER SYSTEMS AND ECOSYSTEMIC THINKING

The idea that it is worthwile to look at and work with an individual, family, and organization in the context of the many larger organizations of which they are a part and the many other organizations with which they interact is becoming increasingly advocated. There is an extensive literature available presenting both ecosystemic thinking and models for working collaboratively with larger systems. Some examples follow.

Adler (in Ansbacher & Ansbacher, 1956) introduced the open forum counseling model shortly after World War I. A referred child was seen with his parents and teachers, in the presence of other parents, teachers and children. The purpose was to normalize difficulties as part of the human condition rather than labeling the child and family as abnormal or sick. Therapist, parents, and child worked together to find understanding and solutions to the problems presented. Since the problem was considered normal, it was also believed that many in the audience would learn from the experience of the group worked with by the therapist. This school/family/ therapist collaboration was considered to be very effective and was implemented in 32 child guidance clinics in Vienna by 1932. Various versions of the open forum counseling method are still very actively used today (Christensen & Schramski, 1983; Kern, Hawes, & Christensen, 1989).

Speck and Atteneave (1973) and Rueveni (1979) described models for including all persons from different systems who might be helpful in sessions with the family. This could include the teacher, clergyman, mailman, neighbors, extended family members, and so on. Meyer proposed an ecosystems approach to social work (1983), advocating that the unit of attention (the patient) be considered within her or his entire world of interactions. Freeman and Pennekamp (1988) describe many ways in which the therapist can extend her arena of practice in reaching out to families, schools, agencies, forming groups of professionals across agencies and disciplines, joining with representatives of multicultural communities, participating in community organizations, and studying with other professionals in lifetime continuous education. They strongly recommend the creation of collaborative relationships across all the demarcated institutional boundaries.

Imber-Black (1988) argues that the therapist can bring together representatives of the various larger systems that impact on the clients to develop and coordinate a larger therapeutic system, including the clients, to help the clients and to reduce the clashing demands of different systems on the clients. The combined effort within a larger therapeutic system that can itself be therapeutically influenced is seen as a major advantage over working solely with the client. Similarly, Stanton and Stanton (1984) present a model in which the therapist can bring together in one room all those actively working with the family—school, community agencies, court workers, clergymen, and others. They allow the expression of competing goals, expectations, wishes, and actions. They thereby dramatize the family's dilemma or impasse and help the family to make decisions that break through the competitive "trajectories" or demands and expectations impacting on them from all these systems.

Some family therapists and family physicians are developing collaborative relationships (*Family Therapy News*, June, 1991). Many other therapists are forming similar collaborations, especially in relation to physical illness, stress, drug abuse, and behavioral medicine. Family therapists and attorneys are working together in relation to divorce counseling and divorce mediation. Forensic psychologists and psychiatrists have long worked as consultants with the court system.

Freeman and Pennekamp (1988) have developed an ecosystemic theory and what they call a shared theoretical map for collaborative interdisciplinary and interorganizational collaboration with the person and the person in environment. They seek to integrate individual, developmental, group, community, and systemic theories and practices.

Silber (1993), with contributions from Lutkes, reports that the National Institute For Mental Health has initiated the Children and Adolescent Service Program (CASSP). This project has stimulated the development of many demonstration programs nationwide to serve mentally ill children. The programs have been based on interagency collaboration to help maintain such children in their homes and schools and out of mental hospitals. The encouraging results of these programs has led in turn to the passage by Congress in 1992 of the so far poorly funded Children's and Communities Mental Health Systems Improvement Act to foster collaborative service delivery systems, including direct work with families. In 1988 the Federation of Families for Children's Mental Health was formed nationally to insist on a parent partnership role in shaping their children's treatment.

Clearly, many professionals, government policy planners, organizations, and lay people are already thinking and practicing collaboratively across disciplines and institutions and thinking about the child and youth in the context of his larger world. Subsequent chapters of this book describe and discuss many concrete examples of collaborative models with families and schools.

IV. INTEGRATING INDIVIDUAL, GROUP, FAMILY, AND SYSTEMS THEORIES

A major advantage of working in collaborative partnerships is that the process almost forces one to begin to find ways of integrating individual psychotherapy theories with systemic theories as the client is considered in the context of his world—particularly in the family and in school as systems. A number of therapists have described in detail integrative models for considering the individual within the system. Among them are Allen (1988), Feldman (1991), Nichols (1987), Sherman and Dinkmeyer (1987), and Wachtel and Wachtel (1986). This movement is driven by the growing recognition among individual therapists that they can no longer ignore the systemic influences on the person; nor can the systems theorists continue to ignore the power of individual motivation and beliefs in the functioning of the human system.

Sherman and Dinkmeyer (1987) observe that the human system is created by individuals acting in concert. When an individual changes behavior, the others in the system must react, often forcing the reorganization of the system. A system is a group of interactive elements organized into a whole. For the organization to work, each part must contribute its piece to the existing whole. However, the organization is built upon a system of rules and roles that guide its operations. Members are influenced to conform to the code by the reciprocal reinforcing behaviors of the other members. This is true whether the system works constructively or destructively, happily or unhappily for its members. Each system in turn is part of larger systems which it influences and by which it is influenced. Therefore, there is always a two-way street of power and influence acting on individual and system. When multiple systems are involved, there is the probability that triangular relationships may emerge that will impact on all.

When two members are engaged in an ongoing conflict, they generally begin on cue and fight in more or less the same pattern and end more or less the same way time after time in a repeating pattern of behavior. The behavior of each calls forth the appropriate reciprocal behavior of the other in a stylized cooperative effort that constitutes their continuing system of fighting. If either refused to cooperate according to the rules in the usual way, the pattern would have to change for better or for worse. Each believes he is doing the only and best thing that he can do under the circumstances.

A child who is not doing his homework may be behaving out of spite to punish parents or teacher for what he perceives as their misbehavior. Or he may believe he isn't good enough—a failure, so what's the use? Or he may be distracting attention from his parents whose fighting threatens the integrity and continuity of the family in the child's eyes. Or maybe father is away most of the time and mother is lonely and angry. When the child misbehaves, mother tells father, who then becomes involved disciplining the child. When father leaves, the child misbehaves again to bring him back into the family joined with mother against the child. The child is in effect a secret ally of mother. In all the above examples, the behavior of the parents reinforces the behavior of the child, thereby maintaining the problem. The problem is not solely in the child's head. A similar pattern is reinforced by the teacher who keeps pressing, ignoring, or punishing the child.

The issue of codependency, especially with respect to alcoholism and addictive behavior, has recently become very popular. Although there are many different definitions of codependency in the literature, the central theme is that people relate with each other reciprocally and complementarily on the basis of their individual needs, thereby reinforcing the problem behavior of the identified client. They wittingly or unwittingly become enablers of the problem behavior. Therefore, the behavior of codependent enablers in relationship with the identified client must be changed in order to facilitate change in the identified client by modifying their patterns of interaction.

A therapist who accepts this kind of integrative picture finds she has greatly increased her options for thinking about the case and for bringing about change. She can examine, challenge, or introduce beliefs and options for the individual, family, school, or peer group within school. She can rearrange the roles of the client and their meanings within the family and school, or she can reorganize all the roles in the systems to change the old repeating patterns. She can change the meanings about self and world and the various objects in that world. She can intervene to block existing dysfunctional patterns of behavior in home or school.

She can reinforce observed strengths and provide many opportunities for personal encouragement within the home and school environment. She can facilitate discussions to evolve constructive common values and goals. She can arrange occasions for the expression of social feeling, belongingness, and concern to overcome feelings of alienation. She can provide for the acquisition of new knowledge and skills to carry forward new ideas and plans. And she can alter the patterns of communication in the home and school through increased awareness, instruction, and interventions in existing patterns. For a detailed description of such a change model see Chapter 1 in Sherman, Oresky, and Rountree (1991).

V. EFFICIENCY AND COST-EFFECTIVENESS

Among the problems with collaborative work are scheduling, the amount of time involved, and cost-effectiveness. The people involved with the child or youth are already involved. Although we have no research data to prove it, we believe from our clinical experience and reports in the literature that working and planning together is more efficient and will save time as a result of more rapid change and less relapse into the same or comparable disturbances.

Obviously, it takes a great deal of time and energy to contact and to find a mutual meeting time and place to bring all the pertinent people together. Secretarial time may be less costly than a professional's time. Having client family members undertake the responsibility may be possible in many cases. Agencies with an outreach department or case managers may be willing to set up the meetings. Once a plan is in place and each person accepts responsibility for his/her part, it may be that no additional meetings are necessary or only one follow-up meeting may be needed. Nevertheless, it is an ambitious undertaking to bring everyone together, to coordinate each person's follow-through, to evaluate and adjust the plan, and to follow-up on progress made.

Rather than attempting the more cumbersome process of bringing *everyone* to the table, for the majority of cases we suggest an effective model that has worked successfully for us—a model that may be more attractive to therapists and more easily accomplished. Because the family and school systems possess the motivation and other properties and advantages described earlier in this chapter, satisfactory creative partnerships with these two institutions may be sufficient to efficiently accomplish our purposes in most cases. Further, a therapist working in a particular local community will tend to have several clients who attend the same schools. Once contacts and mutual trust have been established, it is relatively easy to arrange consultations on subsequent cases. School personnel will probably choose such a therapist for additional referrals. Similarly, a therapist working closely with the school will acquire a reputation among the parents that will facilitate involving the family in the therapeutic process. The therapist and school staff are required to maintain confidentiality, but parents and children do sometimes talk and share with other parents and children about their own experiences.

For children involved with the courts or other social agencies, it may be necessary to join with all concerned parties for the sake of coordination and effectiveness.

A school-based family therapy clinic has the built-in advantage of being connected to the child, the family and to school resources and the mission of combining their joint resources. Such school-based clinics will be described and discussed in Chapter 4.

VI. ISSUES AND CONCERNS IN COLLABORATIVE TREATMENT

Obviously, working collaboratively adds complexity to the treatment process. Although there are many advantages, a number of issues arise that require the attention of the participants. Among them are issues of power, ethics, confidentiality, record keeping, "territoriality," credit and accountability for success, financial arrangements, case responsibility, and liability. How does one combine the efforts of different institutional missions, cultures, languages, styles, time constraints, and even measures of success?

In general, by limiting the partnership to child, family, school, and therapist, and setting the therapist up as the coordinator of the treatment process, many of the problems associated with the above issues are reduced in scope.

A. Power

Power includes who is in charge, how decisions are made, what behaviors are actually enacted and with what results. We suggest that the therapist take the initiative, coordinate the effort, and take responsibility for the overall conduct of the case. However, being the leader/coordinator/facilitator doesn't mean that the therapist makes all the decisions. In this kind of partnership decisions are developed by consensus. Decisions are less likely to work if all parties do not execute their agreed upon commitments. Information and ideas come from all participants. Just as when therapist and individual meet and create a new therapeutic system, so it can be when the therapist brings in the family or convenes a meeting with family and school staff. She can function as a consultant or as a therapist in such a meeting. Both types of models are described in Chapter 3. People take power by doing whatever they do. Each person in the group will exercise power through his/her own actions and those actions in turn will influence the therapeutic system. Therefore, it is essential for the therapist to engage and join with each member.

A major problem may ensue if there is a competition for who is to be in charge. A school principal might fancy him or herself as the one in charge, or one of the parents may be accustomed to that role. This is not an unusual event in therapy. The therapist has many choices. The following are a few of them. The therapist can deliberately move into a one-down position, thus making herself nonthreatening while simultaneously taking therapeutic steps. She can move into the role of consultant to the group, allowing it to be "chaired" by another. (See Schmidt [1993, Chapter 6] for a consultation model that can be used in working with school and family.) She can describe what is going on to the group and make it a decision-making choice as to how the group wants to handle the leadership function. She can point out that this is a therapy session convened by her and she is the therapist. The best choice is a creative decision, which is dictated by the circumstances.

In terms of power in the family and defusing and redirecting the power play in family therapy, the reader is referred to Sherman (1983) and Sherman, Oresky, and Rountree (1991, Chapter 12), and Nichols and Deissler (1988).

B. Ethics, Confidentiality, and Record Keeping

The first problem is whose code of ethics will be observed when members of different professions are involved. Fortunately, there is a great deal of overlap among the various codes with the best interest of the client always the principal concern. If an ethical question arises, it should be discussed among the professionals with the best interest of the client as the guide for making an informed decision. If it is a serious matter, the members can consult with their various ethics boards. If there is a question of law, such as reporting child abuse to the proper authorities, then the action taken will conform with the law. If law and ethics are in dispute, such as in cases of client confidentiality versus reporting, then it is up to the conscience of the therapist, who must be prepared to take the consequences of her decision. Most professions assume that law will prevail unless and until it is changed, perhaps through political activism.

When the client is being seen by multiple parties, such as school counselor, teacher, and therapist, or the therapist sees the family for some sessions separately from school staff, it is quite likely that information will be given in such meetings. It is helpful to seek agreement at the beginning that all information may be considered shared at the discretion of the professionals, unless specifically enjoined by another participant that this piece of information is confidential. If the therapist or the receiver of the information thinks it is important, then part of the work is to discuss the need to share this information with other members. Examples of permission forms are to be found in Appendix A.

Secrets generally sustain the client and systemic problem and make change more difficult. It is better to eliminate as many secrets as possible. There are exeptions, of course. One phrase often heard relative to the sharing of information is "on an as-needed basis." This gives a great deal of power to the holder of the information. Again, usually, the more that is shared, the more effective each partner in the process can be. The more open the system, the more likely is it to change.

Ethically and morally we seek permission to share information among the members. It is necessary to prepare written permission forms and have these signed by the clients to permit sharing among a fixed circle of participants and separate forms if others need to be informed or solicited for information such as for medical reports.

One issue in record keeping concerns which individuals other than the direct members of the treatment group will have access to the records. Another is will family members have access to the records? Court cases have provided considerable access to school records by parents, generally including noncustodial parents. Most ethical codes allow cooperating professionals to share information in the service of the child. But who else in a cooperating organization can obtain the file? Licensed psychologists and psychiatrists, physicians, lawyers, and clergymen typically possess some degree of confidentiality before the law. School staff do not have such privileges. Other mental health professionals, such as counselors and marriage and family therapists, sometimes do not have such privileges. These are determined by the laws in each state separately.

Agencies with externally funded programs will have to submit reports to their oversight evaluators. This often includes case files. Insurance carriers may also demand a copy of the record or a detailed report.

It is likely that both therapist and one or more school staff members will keep records on the case consonant with their respective roles and each will protect the confidentiality of the records consistent with law and ethics.

Should there be a malpractice suit or if records are legally required by the courts for any reason, it is expected that the therapist's records will minimally include a diagnostic statement, a treatment plan, progress notes, dates of meetings, and who was in attendance.

If sessions are to be recorded on audio or videotape, all participants must be informed and sign consent agreements, which include the purpose to which the recordings will be put. For example, they will be used for educational training of professionals, to share with other collaborators, to be shown to the family so the members can observe how they behave, or to be available for sale commercially.

C. Responsibility, Liability, and Accountability

Even though the therapist may undertake the initiative of coordinating the case and facilitating an overall treatment plan, each part of the treatment system retains responsibility for itself. The clients are responsible for their behavior; the parents for parenting; the therapist for the therapy; and the school for schooling. Each professional is liable for malpractice. Parents are accountable for abuse or neglect. All are responsible for carrying out their part of the treatment plan agreed upon.

Short of malpractice, there are in fact few elements of accountability in place for the professionals involved. If dissatisfied with the process, the child or family have the power to increase their level of resistance, withdraw from the therapy, move to another school district, place the child in a private school, or complain to higher authority. If the therapist finds the school too rigid, she can only work therapeutically with the system in hopes of modifying its patterns. Under some circumstances she might choose to take on an advocacy role on behalf of the client or family. Such a choice may create conflict within the collaborative team. Similarly, if the family is dysfunctional, the therapist will use family therapy techniques to bring about changes in the family system.

The beauty of working collaboratively is that it brings all the elements together in a new system. This new system contains both additional options in an expanded system that were previously not available and new checks and balances on all the participants to help keep them more on target.

Each part of the collaborative sytem may come with different goals. For example, the children may consider the program successful if parents and teachers get off their backs. The school may consider the program successful if the child is behaving in class, doing homework, and getting reasonable grades. The therapist may be looking for the child to acquire a better sense of self-esteem and achieve greater separation-individuation in the family system.

Clearly, the team has to devise common goals that will somehow incorporate these subsystem goals. For example, do all the participants wish for a more friendly and cooperative pattern of interacting with each other? If so, could one subgoal be that parents and teachers will nag and criticize less while the child will assume more responsibility for homework and chores? Could the child be asked to identify where and how she or he needs help and where not? Other subgoals could address other issues recognizing the complementarity of the interactive patterns of behavior.

D. Financial Arrangements

Both independent practitioners and most agencies expect to be paid for their services based on their fee schedules. School staffs, especially in the public schools, do not yet charge extra for additional services, such as testing and counseling and meetings with parents and therapist. If the clients are privately insured or funded through Medicaid or some other insurance program, fees need to be worked out with the family in terms of the insurance provisions and stated fee schedules of the therapist.

Medicare and Medicaid make it clear that the therapist must accept assignment plus coinsurance of a stated approved amount. Some therapists will attend a limited number of family-school meetings and engage in a limited number of necessary telephone calls pro bono. Others insist on payment, rating each meeting as one session. Still others insist on being paid for as many sessions as such meetings and calls would equate to in hours. All such arrangements must be negotiated in advance so there can be no misunderstanding of what was agreed to. It is understood that if third-party payments are involved, the claim cannot be fraudulently misstated to conform to the terms of the insurance policy.

E. Dealing with Different Missions and Cultures

Just as each person or subgroup may have its own goals, each also comes with its own mythology, beliefs, expectations, language, and ways of doing things. The therapist, family, and school have somewhat different missions in our society and different visions and styles as to how to carry out those missions. For example, there are dramatic differences in democratic versus authoritarian child-rearing methods or punishment versus positive reinforcement as ways of developing new behavior. In this heterogeneous society, individual families, schools, and therapists create their own ways.

Think of how many different systems of individual and family therapy there are, each with its own emphases and vocabulary! One of the authors was scheduled to speak to all the support staff of the many high schools of a large urban school district. Preceding the talk the group held a business meeting. The author was utterly dumbfounded and had no idea what these clinicians were talking about using their own abbreviations and systems designs, in spite of his wide acqaintance with many schools over many years and knowing personally some of the staff in the group. One can imagine that some children and parents would also have difficulty learning the language and ways of a given school.

The same is true for school professionals and therapists who have to learn the multicultures and languages of the families and children they deal with. The authors observe that even children in a given school and neighborhood develop new languages, fads, fashions, and world views at the rate of about every two years in the high schools and colleges and slightly more slowly in the lower grades. This is particularly true in rapidly changing neighborhoods.

Such differences and rapid changes create formidable tasks for the collaborative team in understanding one another and their respective systems. Therefore, it is important to question the meaning of even common words and how things are done. One parent said that her 12-year-old daughter reported that she was going steady with a boy. When the girl was asked what that means she replied that she sits with him in English and social studies classes. Most of us would have leaped to some other conclusions, as did the girl's mother. The news media recently reported the case of hardworking, well-regarded parents who had chained up their 15-year-old daughter in the family living room "to protect her" from taking crack cocaine. Many neighbors who were interviewed were appalled, although some thought it was probably appropriate and in the girl's best interest. The girl herself supported the parents.

The therapist needs to use all her powers of empathy, a healthy curiousity about the other members of the collaborative team and the school, and a willingness to let the others teach her about themselves. She needs to create an atmosphere of mutual acceptance and respect. She will use all her skills for developing rapport and joining. She will stimulate a willingness among all to negotiate differences and come to mutual agreements.

F. Territoriality

Territoriality involves issues of control, inclusion and exclusion, and boundaries. It cuts across many of the issues previously discussed. What is my responsibility and what is yours?
Who pays for this and who collects for that? Who gets blame
or credit? Who is "rightfully" in charge or who is "obligated"
to be in charge or to coordinate? Whose job is a given aspect
of the treatment plan? Sometimes a given worker or agency
wants to take on more or avoid more of the work or
responsibility.

Most workers and agencies have a clear sense of their mission and professional competencies. When the team members are mutually respectful of one another's positions and
missions, they are usually able to negotiate the issues of turf
or territoriality.

The rewards of working collaboratively far outweigh the
increased complexity of the process. One of the greatest rewards is that the therapist can see the principal players in
action on the scene rather than having to rely on reported
data as perceived by the individual client alone. She can therefore design a more realistic therapeutic plan by interacting
with all the players and thus bring about constructive change.
Hopefully, by changing both the individuals and the systems
involved, the changes will be less susceptible to relapse or to
the substitution of a new dysfunctional symptom to replace
the old one because the system still requires some form of
symptomatic behavior to maintain itself. For example, correcting the misbehavior of one child who is acting out, to
keep mother active and mobilized so that she does not suc-
cumb to overwhelming depression, may lead to the acting
out behavior of another sibling unless something is done to
assist mother's depressed position in the family. Her depression may serve to convert her husband's rage and impending
violence into sympathy and caringness. The therapist looks
at and acts upon the total picture.

Chapters 8 and 9 provide two detailed case studies in which
such issues are discussed and resolved by the participants.

CHAPTER 2

WHAT THERAPISTS MIGHT FIND IN SCHOOLS

A. OVERVIEW

Blaming and cross blaming have become a national preoccupation. Each administration blames the earlier one for its problems; our TV screens project endless police and courtroom scenes dealing with the "who done it" question; huge sums of money are being collected in insurance compensation if appropriate blame can be proved by a victim.

Blaming and cross blaming have been part of human nature since time immemorial. God blames Adam, who blames his wife, who blames the serpent for man's tragic existence. Droughts, floods, and disease were often blamed on an individual culprit or a small group of transgressors. Since humans have been interested in issues of "right" and "wrong," in villains and victims, they have been seeking the source of blame and the chance to even out the scales of justice.

Certain developments in the pattern of blaming have occurred over the decades. Before the rise of the age of science and reason with its emphasis on individual responsibility, blame for social and natural mishaps was attributed to the sins of a few. Our present society seems to have reversed the emphasis. We tend to focus more on institutional, organizational, and the total social context as the source of the ills of the individual. Thus the schools are blamed for children's failure to learn; the family for children's emotional problems; the workplace for mental instability; the "economy" for individual crimes.

Although all these attributions have a degree of validity, one should question the effectiveness of investing so much of our emotional and cognitive energy in finger pointing rather than in problem solving.

Schools and families are not free of the blaming–cross blaming attitude. A practitioner who works with a family whose child is having psychological symptoms often hears comments and convictions such as these: "My 15-year-old began the 5th grade when he had a teacher who didn't understand him." "I don't want to be called into school anymore. They created the problem. Let them deal with it." "My child doesn't belong in special education. She is placed there because her teachers don't know how to teach."

Blaming is rampant in the other direction. Children's problems at school are blamed on a variety of family crimes and misdemeanors: divorce, poverty, lack of appropriate parenting skills, drug abuse, physical and sexual abuse, ignorance, or cultural heritage.

Such factors affecting children's lives must not be ignored. However, pinning responsibility often fails to move into a more productive problem-solving stage.

The application of systems theory to human behavior is instrumental in attempting to reduce a blaming orientation. Viewing behavior in the context of its total interactive system shifts the focus from the victim-villain equation to a circular perspective where all parts of the system participate in a reciprocal manner. Children's dysfunctional behavior is therefore seen as part of a more comprehensive pattern of behavior affecting the total family and/or school.

Systemic and ecological concepts that helped broaden the understanding of family interaction only recently have been applied to families in the context of larger systems. Elizur & Minuchin (1990) are among those who have moved in this direction in describing the development of pathological symptoms as part of the institutionalization context. They demonstrate the role of the structure of an organization such as a hospital in exacerbating pathology in an individual and his or her family. Patricia Minuchin (1992) has been working on applying a family-community systems model to welfare and foster-care families.

Weiss and Edwards at the Ackerman Institute have devised a model of school consultation based on a school-family collaborative macro system (1992). Imber-Black (1988) in her study of families in the larger context of multiple services has also contributed to the understanding of family functioning as related to larger system context. Lusterman places school-family interaction in the context of a larger system, which he describes in terms of an ecomap (1985/1988). A number of such models will be described in detail in Chapter 3. It is helpful for the therapist to become familiar with the structure of schools and classrooms in order to better collaborate with the school and the family .

This chapter is devoted to an exploration of the school-family collaboration from two perspectives:

1. The view that a school system is a living organization that can be understood by application of family system concepts.
2. The view that family-school interaction is not only a function of two separate interacting systems, but that they are part of a larger macrosystem that provides a context for a significant portion of the child's experience.

B. HOW SCHOOLS ARE ORGANIZED AS A SYSTEM

The child's school world can be viewed as a series of concentric circles that constitute the various subsystems of the educational context. Some of these subsystems are small and immediate. The classroom is an example of such a sub-system where the child interacts directly with teachers and peers. The potential for classroom teacher and family collaboration is high, and contact between therapist and teacher is most essential.

A larger and less immediate circle might be a given level within a school building (e.g., grade level, or elementary, secondary, or preschool levels). A less immediate subsystem is the services component in a school building. These services include guidance, school psychology, and social work, remedial programs, special-education resource-room instruction, special programs for the gifted, and other supportive services. They are essentially pull-out programs serving students in individual or small groups. Contact between students and service personnel is rather intimate, though less frequent. Communication between service personnel and families is often built into policies defining these services.

The building administrative and supervisory subsystem is another step further removed from direct contact with student and family. This group includes principals, assistant principals, program directors, and coordinators. Although noncompliance and discipline problems often bring administration into direct contact with students and their families, most contact tends to be indirect. Their impact on students and families is channeled through their effect on school climate, policies, and quality of communication with teaching and service staff. However, these individuals are important for the therapist to know and to work with, as they often have the power to facilitate desirable changes in the student's school program, the school climate affecting the child, and communication patterns within the school.

The central administrative and supervisory subsystem (superintendent, assistant superintendent, central curriculum director, director of pupil services) have minimal direct contact with children and their families but carry enormous weight in setting the stage for school-family collaboration. Programs in parent education, parent participation, and staff development opportunities designed to increase collaboration are all highly instrumental in developing and sustaining a close relationship between the school and its clientele, namely, the student, parents and community. Therapists can play an extremely important role as consultants to central administrators in setting up collaboration programs as well as in participating in the training of school personnel in developing communications skills and enhancing school-family collaboration.

Further removed from direct contact with students and parents, yet extremely influential, are central governmental bodies dealing with education. These include central boards of education in large cities, state education departments, federal agencies, and the courts. Although the relationship between these organizations and the daily lives of children and parents is not obvious, it is nevertheless very powerful. For example, the passage of Federal Public Law 94-142 has had a major impact on individual school systems and all their various subsystems. This law mandates appropriate education for all handicapped children in a least-restrictive environment, which affords disabled children opportunities to intermingle and share educational experiences with nonimpaired students.

The implementation of multicultural curricula initiated at state levels is having a significant impact on local programs designed to develop a positive self-image in diverse minority pupils and their families. Hopefully, such programs will succeed in empowering children and parents of minorities.

The role of the therapist in affecting interaction between such governmental bodies and individual families may be minimal. However, the therapist may impact on them through a political or consultative involvement.

It is helpful for the therapist to become familiar with the structure of the classroom and other school subsystems in order to better collaborate with the school and the family and to facilitate collaboration between them.

1. The Classroom as a Subsystem

As a living social organization, the classroom shares certain characteristics with other social systems. It has boundaries within and around it and these may vary in their degree of clarity and flexibility. It can also be viewed in terms of cohesion, hierarchical organization, power distribution, patterns of communication, and other criteria used in describing interactions within living social systems.

a. The Cohesion-Differentiation Continuum

Cohesion refers to interactional patterns that encourage togetherness and support, whereas differentiation refers to empowerment of individuality and independence within the group. A balance between these factors would appear to be most beneficial for the group and the individual, although extremes at both ends of the continuum may result in dysfunction. At one extreme of the cohesion continuum are classrooms that stress conformity in thinking and conduct as well as homogeneity in achievement and perspective. These characteristics may be achieved by benevolent and supportive means or by an imposing authoritarian style. Either way, teacher control and structure dominate the scene whereas individual differences in ability, interest, and background are not given their due recognition.

At the other extreme are classrooms lacking in cohesion. They tend to have a very loose structure and a minimal sense of togetherness. Teacher control may be poor, expectations ambiguously communicated, instructions may be unclear or contradictory although conflict among individuals is high. Children are expected to make independent decisions for which they are unprepared. This situation may border on the chaotic.

The classroom in the middle range is characterized by feelings of togetherness, group pride, teacher support, and mutual support among students, allowing for appropriate expression of conflict and competition. Although instructions and expectations are clearly communicated, there is room for student input, negotiation, and planning. Empathy and support are evident between teacher and students as well as within the peer group. Differences are respected.

b. Role Hierarchy

Concepts of role hierarchy and power distribution are as applicable to classroom dynamics as they are to family process. They will be discussed here under the concept of the authoritarian versus permissive teaching style continuum.

At the authoritarian extreme of the continuum, one finds classrooms where boundaries and hierarchies between teachers and students are rather fixed and rigid. The teacher's position at the highest point in the hierarchy is rarely questioned. Decision-making power is totally in his or her hands. The teacher determines the content and sequence of the lessons with little or no input from students. The teacher determines rules for behavior which students must follow. Students usually engage in the same activity simultaneously. Practice and repetition are highly stressed.

Although few classrooms of this nature represent an acceptable model in the mainstream of American education today, it is not totally absent. It does represent a familiar and thus acceptable model to parents who have experienced such schools in the past or those who were exposed to authoritarian models of education in other countries.

At the other extreme of the continuum are classrooms in which role hierarchies are blurred and insufficient power is imbued in the teacher and an inappropriate degree of power and direction is given to students. Students tend to sway the teacher's direction and often derail discussion from the central focus. Scheduling is poorly adhered to while the teacher's feedback is inconsistent and unclear. Because of the inappropriate distribution of power, such classrooms are also characterized by weak boundaries and a tendency to be chaotic.

At the middle range of the continuum are classrooms where hierarchical relationships are well defined and power appropriately distributed. The adult (parent, teacher) clearly occupies an authority position, but lines of communication between the hierarchies are open and circular. Student views and preferences are seriously taken into account while the final decision-making power and leadership lie with the teacher. Students are empowered by actively participating in the learning process and by being respected for their uniqueness. However, roles are clearly established and are appropriately empowered.

c. Triadic Relationships

Triadic relationships with their variations have been extensively described in the family therapy research literature by Bowen (1978), Minuchin (1974), and Haley (1976). This concept deals with issues of closeness, distance, alliances, coalitions, loyalties, and the intensity of emotional investment between and within members of the family.

The organization of a school building and the classroom within it can be viewed as a series of interlocking triangles. Among the most obvious examples of common triangles within a school organization are the parent-teacher-student triangle; the student-student-teacher triangle; the administration-student-teacher triangle; the classroom teacher-service personnel-student triangle. Two examples that demonstrate triangular relationships within the school organization will be discussed.

The parent-teacher-student triangle has a number of possible variations. Parent and student may form an alliance, keeping the teacher in an "outside" position. For example, parents may support their child's contention that a failure on a test or a poor grade is due to the teacher's unfair grading system; or a parent may keep a child at home to care for younger siblings and the child is asked to withhold from the teacher the true reason for the absence. Or, a child may develop a school avoidance problem as a means of warding off parental divorce or depression and the teacher is blamed for the child's problem.

Another common triangle is one in which parent and teacher form an alliance, keeping the student in an "outside" position. For example, parent and teacher devise a tight supervision plan to make sure that the student completes his or her homework, while the student remains resistant to the efforts of both parent and teacher. Another example is when a parent requests a teacher to administer disciplinary action to control the child's behavior at home.

A student-teacher alliance with parent in an "outside" position is also fairly common. For instance, a teacher fails to report to parents about the student's misbehavior, fearing parent retaliation toward the child. This level of triangulation also may be present when a child gains concessions from a teacher due to the latter's sympathy over harshness, neglect, deprivation, and abuse on the part of the parent.

Awareness of such dynamics is extremely important for the mental health practitioner. Although the issues involved may have a realistic base (child abuse, teacher rigidity, excessive punitiveness on the part of the school or the family), the practitioner can help tease out reality issues from emotional biases and reduce the levels of distance between the parties. He or she can help create triangles of equidistance focused on problem solving. Meeting together with parents, teacher, and student, the practitioner can facilitate communication regarding expectations and means of achieving them.

Student-student-teacher triangle may involve one adult and two or more children. This may occur in a classroom where a power struggle exists between teacher and students. Students may form an alliance to negate teacher authority. Or, a teacher may try to separate students and break a close friendship to "protect" one student from the "negative influence" of the other. An uneven triangular alliance may also be evident when a teacher "adopts" a child as helper, often causing distance between this student and his peers.

Such triangles often resemble the parent-siblings triangles. Siblings may form a coalition to gain power in a conflictual relationship with the parent (assisting a sibling to carry out an action forbidden by the parent, or keeping secrets concerning the sibling's transgression). A parent may "select" a child as a partner, causing closeness between the parent and child or conflict or distance with other siblings.

Helping teachers increase their awareness of such interaction may bring greater objectivity and reduce the emotional pull toward triangulation. School-based family-oriented mental health practitioners as well as private agencies can play an important role in facilitating such awareness. This can occur on an individual consultation basis or as part of a larger professional development program.

2. The Family and the Classroom as Interactive System

Children spend most of their waking hours between the classroom and the family. These settings may be conceived as two parts of a larger system in which the child functions. The independent therapist or agency- and school-based mental health personnel need to be aware not only of the dynamics within each setting, but also the dynamics of the interactions between them. The need to assume this perspective arises when questions such as these occur:

- Why does a given student do well in one grade and poorly in another?
- When a "troublemaker" is removed from the classroom to a special program, why does another student often emerge as the next "troublemaker"?
- Do parents misrepresent or distort reality when they deny that problems evident in the classroom are not evident at home?

The answers to such questions may be found in studying each context separately, but more fruitfully, perhaps, in studying the interaction between each of these environments as a microsystem of a larger family-home macrosystem.

Case Example: When Authority and Boundaries Differ

Tina's family had recently immigrated to the U.S. from the Caribbean. Her parents are both employed and are working hard to maintain the intactness of their family. They have both had an elementary school education fashioned after a European colonial model in which the teacher's authority is unquestioned and student participation occurs only in response to the teacher's demand. Tina had attended four grades in this type of school. When she entered the 5th grade in the U.S., she confronted a school environment where she was expected to work independently, work with other students on group projects, and speak up in front of other students. The shift between the two school environments and the continuing difference between the interactions at home and those at school presented problems for her. She failed to make appropriate academic progress because of her inability to assume initiative and responsibility for her work. Furthermore, she began to "act up" because she often interpreted her teacher's informality and openness as weakness. A conference between Tina's mother and her teacher increased the gap between the school and the parent. Although Tina's mother felt that the teacher was "too easy" on her child, the teacher felt that the family was too rigid, lacking in empathy, and holding unreasonable and narrow expectations for their child.

The mental health practitioner's intervention brought the teacher, student, and family together. She encouraged self-expression at both ends and validated the perspective of each. Each participant was empowered by being labeled "hard working" and "caring." Tina was labeled as a good student who is continuing to act as if she were still in her old school. Differences were labeled as cultural rather than personal. Departure from one "true" method was urged and each side was encouraged to adopt some of the characteristics of the other. The teacher was encouraged to give Tina more specific structure and instruction, while helping Tina take small steps in learning to think and work more independently. The family was urged to introduce appropriate choice-making opportunities and small modifications in hierarchical boundaries, giving Tina a chance to participate in decisions concerning her activities. Tina was urged to help the teacher and parents move in these directions.

CASE EXAMPLE: WHEN SIBLING POSITIONS DIFFER

Ross, an 8-year-old boy, is the oldest of three children. His two younger brothers are 6 and 2. Ross is relatively large for his age. He is also an excellent student and is highly verbal and knowledgeable. However, Ross has social problems at school. He is not well liked by his peers and therefore has no friends. Feeling that nobody likes him, he makes no attempt to reach out and make friends. Contact between the therapist and the classroom teacher followed by a field observation revealed the following:

Ross is the first to know the answer to the teacher's questions. He calls out his answers without being asked. This angers the teacher and other children who are deprived of their chance to respond. This behavior continues in spite of reminders and private talks with the teacher. On the playground and at lunch, Ross is engaged in frequent criticism of other children, moralizing or offering opinions about what is right. The children tend to ignore him or respond with ridicule. At games, he is one of the last to be selected on teams. He reacts with anger and challenge to the leaders for not doing things correctly. He is a stickler for rules and doesn't let a deviation go unchallenged. This behavior pattern, which does not endear him socially, is not responsive to intervention by school personnel.

The picture becomes clearer when the family constellation is brought into focus.

Ross's parents are both first born. Their first child is therefore the oldest of a whole generation of cousins. He is admired by the adults in the family for his brightness and adultlike behavior. At family gatherings, he is the undisputed leader. However, he prefers adult company to that of his siblings and "baby cousins."

The two pictures represent discrepancies between the family's perception of his behavior as "mature" and the perception of his school behavior by teachers and peers as "one-upmanship."

The therapist working with both parts of the system can help bring about collaboration, cross communication and bridging of the expectations for Ross at school and at home. The therapist can help the school understand Ross in terms of his family context, while helping the family set clearer boundaries between the child and adult hierarchies.

3. Organization of the Support Services Subsystem and the Family

School support services consist of a variety of specialists offering remedial or enrichment services usually in small groups outside the classroom setting. They include guidance counselors at the elementary and secondary levels; school psychologists, resource-room teachers; remedial reading and math teachers; nurses; teachers for the gifted; and social workers and specialists for the hearing, visually, and physically impaired.

The relationship between these services is horizontal rather than hierarchical. They usually operate as a team in each school building. Relationship with the classroom teacher is also nonhierarchical. In a collaborative school climate, the service team and teachers work closely together. In the absence of such a climate, they tend to become competitive. A hierarchical relationship exists among service personnel, building, and central administrators.

Most of these services are provided through the Committee on Special Education (CSE). Although not all students seen by therapists receive services under the umbrella of special education, a brief examination of the type of handicapping conditions covered by special education services suggests that a large proportion of students with problems are likely to be involved with CSE. These include autistic; emotionally disturbed; learning disabled; speech and language impaired; mentally retarded; deaf and hard of hearing, blind and visually impaired; and the physically impaired.

Although a certain proportion of students such as the failing, underachieving, truant, school-phobic, acting-out, the shy, or isolated receive services outside the umbrella of special education, a detailed examination of this program provides a useful model for all other service programs. Of particular interest to mental health practitioners are not only the resources made available through the Committee, but also the specific ways in which families participate throughout the referral-evaluation-implementation and review processes. The potential for family-school collaboration inherent in the legal aspects of special education can serve as a model for collaboration in family-school service relationships around the needs of those who are not classified as "handicapped." With the legal constraints removed, it can offer flexibility for professionals interested in facilitating school-family interaction. Let us first examine some of the legal aspects.

a. Public Law 94-142 and 99-457

Public Law 94-142, signed in 1975, mandates free and appropriate education for individuals with handicapping conditions in a least-restrictive environment. This law, originally pertaining to school-age children, was recently amended (PL 99-457) to include preschool children. Appropriate educational services must be individually designed and closely monitored. Evaluations must be nondiscriminatory and must be conducted in the student's primary language. Schools must include parents in decisions concerning the evaluation, placement, program, and follow-up of their children. Parents are entitled to "due-process" hearings to help resolve differences with school recommendations.

b. The Referral Process

Students suspected of having a handicapping condition are expected to be referred for a full psychoeducational evaluation. The referral process usually begins at a school building level where the need for this step is assessed by a building team. This group is usually comprised of teachers, counselors, administrator, school psychologist, and other professionals involved with the student's program. A student believed to require further study is referred to the Committee on Special Education (CSE). It is important to note that an independent therapist could also refer a child for study with parent permission.

Referral for an evaluation requires parental approval. A description of the procedures to be undertaken as well as information concerning parents' rights are given to the parent at the inception of the referral process. The major effort involved at this juncture, however, extends beyond these procedural steps. The nature of the contact at this point often determines whether schools and families will work together or grow apart.

Most parents receive the news concerning the referral as a threat. Although school personnel may invest much effort in helping reduce parental anxiety, it is extremely difficult to spare parents the pain involved. Since referral is based on a perceived deviation from a general norm, it usually signifies to the parents that the child is failing or is different from other children. It is a rare parent who can separate his or her own sense of self-worth from the degree of success or failure experienced by the child. A child's "failure," more often than not, is translated in the parents' mind into their failure as parents and people or the school's failure. Thus, the blaming process may quickly emerge. The legal language used in communicating with parents ("due process," "right to appeal") further increases anxiety, suspiciousness, and polarization.

The school may unwittingly contribute to the communication gap. Due to insufficient familiarity with the workings of specific families or with general dynamics of family functioning, educators tend to misjudge anxiety for lack of cooperation. For example, a mother who refuses to give permission for the child's testing may be reflecting reluctance on the part of other key members of the family (e.g., husband or grandparent). She may feel that she is betraying her own mother by producing a "damaged" child; or she may feel that members of the extended family will hold her responsible for the problem. School personnel who are not aware of such underlying feelings may label the parent "resistant," "uncooperative," "disinterested," or "overprotective." Such attitudes may be subtly communicated to the parent, thus increasing the gap in family-school collaboration.

Mental health professionals, whether they are school-based or operate independently, can be of great assistance in reducing the gap. By bringing school personnel and parents together with a third party (therapist), both sides can develop greater understanding of each other's position, identify areas of concern, and arrive at an acceptable solution.

On a private level, a practitioner can help families become more familiar with the process and gain a better view of the advantages inherent in taking the step. Private practitioners are particularly suited for this role because they tend to be perceived by parents as members of their own team. The fact that no action can be taken by the Committee without parental consent needs to be emphasized. Awareness of this level of control on the part of the family often reduces anxiety and suspiciousness.

c. The Evaluation Process

A full assessment undertaken under the auspices of the Committee on Special Education includes cognitive measures, a physical examination, educational achievement status, and other tests designed to probe for specific problems, such as learning disabilities, language deficits, attention deficits, emotional handicaps, or perceptual problems. It also includes a psychosocial history, which covers developmental history and family background.

With the exception of the psychosocial history, most tests take place between a professional and a child, excluding parents from the process.

Bringing the family into the evaluation process can enrich the understanding of children as learners and supply a broader context to information yielded by tests or classroom observations.

How does the family interview enhance and complement the evaluation conducted by means of diagnostic tests?

The interaction between a mental health professional and the family can offer rich data concerning the cognitive aspects of the child's behavior. For instance, a child who is diagnosed as having "expressive language deficit" may be traditionally assumed to "own" the deficit. A family interview may pose these possibilities: that the child is reacting to a highly volatile situation where clear and direct communication is not generally practiced, or the child may be mirroring a communication system where little is being said or expected to be said among members of the family. Variations on the theme of communication patterns in the family and their impact on children's language development are infinite but they do have a way of surfacing to an observable level when the family and child are seen in a system context.

Behaviors generally described as "attention deficit" or "lack of organization" can likewise be interpreted as a function of a deficit inherent in the child or as a function of the family system. Seeing the family together may reveal poor organization in the family in many aspects of its functioning (time and space arrangements, rules, roles, and boundaries). An "attention" deficit may be a part of a larger family communication pattern characterized by poor listening, distractibility, or insufficient feedback. (The relationship between learning patterns and family dynamics will be discussed in greater detail in Chapter 6.)

Social and emotional problems defined as a dysfunction within the child can also be examined from a family perspective. A whole host of attitudes and behavior patterns, such as attitudes toward achievement, frustration tolerance, attitudes toward authority, and issues of trust and self-confidence, may all be better understood in the context of family interactions.

The completion of a psychosocial history, an evaluation procedure mandated by law, comes close to an evaluative technique that brings school personnel and parent into direct contact. It is designed to obtain information concerning the student's physical, cognitive, and social development as well as facts concerning the family constellation. It provides useful information as to *what* occurs in the family but offers little insight into family processes, which are the *how* of family functioning. A psychosocial evaluation can offer more complete data through the utilization of family interview techniques.

The use of family systems interviews should not be used as a substitute for individual intelligence, motor-visual perception, language, or personality evaluative measurements. It is proposed as a broader perspective offering a view of process and context that cannot be obtained through standard diagnostic means.

Families can be greatly empowered by their participation in the evaluation process. As adults who are most familiar with the child, they can be included in the process as a valuable resource. It is only when school personnel are able to give up their "teaching" role toward parents and parents feel that they add a valuable dimension to the school's view of the child that productive collaboration can take place.

Therapists working with families outside the school setting can enhance the collaborative effort in a number of ways. With parental permission, they can share relevant information concerning family process as well as individual concerns and provide their insights to school support personnel. They can also make recommendations based on these insights, support the family, and help reduce undue anxiety, thus facilitating greater trust and receptivity on both sides.

d. The Family and the Committee on Special Education

Upon completion of the student evaluation, a meeting is held between the Committee and the family. The Committee consists of various school professionals and a parent of a handicapped child in the district. When appropriate, the student under consideration is also present. Parents must be informed of the meeting date and invited to attend. The parents are asked for their input and have a right to accept or reject the recommendations of the Committee. The meeting is designed to achieve two objectives: classify the student according to the diagnostic classifications outlined in Public Law 94-142 and develop an Individual Educational Plan (IEP) that addresses issues of placement, support services, curriculum, special equipment, transportation, and other needs.

Both of these issues are emotionally loaded and therefore subject to miscommunication, defensive posturing, and a reduced problem-solving potential.

Diagnostic classifications such as "mental retardation," "emotional disturbance," "learning disability," or "speech and language impairment" carry an extremely threatening message. They conjure up certain images in a parent's mind: ostracism by peers, neighbors, and extended family, as well as ridicule and isolation. Parents further fear the detrimental impact on the child's self-image and the self-fulfilling prophecy associated with labeled classification. In addition to such realistic concerns, there is often another layer of anxiety in parents. It is the search for failure in themselves as an explanation for their child's deficit.

Labeling can also have a liberating effect on students, teachers, and families. When a child's problem is attributed to a disability rather than willful resistance, laziness, lack of responsibility, or lack of family support, pressure is eased. However, in spite of its liberating potential, the process of classification is wrought with a great deal of anguish for most families.

It is not surprising that school service personnel often find themselves at odds with families on this issue. Although therapists are tuned into such issues and can help people with divergent positions find a common solution, they also find themselves in a dilemma around the issue of classification. The school, as represented by the Committee on Special Education, tends to follow the medical model by assigning diagnoses to individual children according to "deficits" inherent in them (e.g., student "has" a disability). The systems-oriented therapist or school-based service professional recognizes the self-fulfilling power of diagnostic labels. Child symptoms are viewed not as an independent entity but as a function of the total family system. Defining the problem as inherent in the child does not only ignore the family-based and school-based facets of the problem, it actively contributes to an intensification of scapegoating.

This issue cannot be resolved through direct exchange with schools or families. It is inherent in the legal formulation of PL 42-149, which schools are mandated to follow. It is an area, however, in which therapists as a group, primarily through their associations, attempt to influence legislative philosophy involved in providing for the educational needs of exceptional children.

The development of the Individual Educational Plan (IEP), the second charge of the Committee on Special Education, poses other emotional challenges for the family and the school. One of the cornerstones of the mandate concerning special education is the concept of "least-restrictive environment." It must always be considered in the development of the IEP. The definition of least restrictive is relative to the nature of the handicapping condition. It represents a range of services from placement in a regular classroom with part-time supportive services, to a self-contained classroom, special day school or a residential placement. Placement in a self-contained class for an autistic child may be least restrictive as it provides educational opportunities in the home community. On the other hand, a mildly retarded child may profit most in a least-restrictive program that consists of partial placement in a self-contained classroom along with participation in nonacademic regular classes.

With the exception of severely and profoundly handicapped children, whose parents may seek a protective environment in a segregated setting, most parents tend to opt for as conventional a program as possible. They tend to prefer resource-room services to self-contained classes, public school-based placement to special schools, and so on. Because the degree of segregation is often associated with the severity of the handicapping condition, it is not surprising that parents perceive placement in less restrictive programs as a hopeful sign. They may find themselves at odds with school personnel who have no emotional investment in minimizing the severity of the handicapping condition.

Another area of potential divergence between the school and the family in determining programs and services occurs around the issue of "appropriate education." Although regulations are relatively clear on issues such as class size or amount and frequency of supportive services, parents and school personnel may differ on the definition of "appropriate education" during the development of the IEP. Parents may wish for more service than the school deems appropriate or may question the efficacy and extent of special services.

Such differences are to be expected. Parents who question and challenge the Committee are often strong advocates for their children. It is the powerless and depressed family that is unable to advocate for its children and thus accepts school recommendations without question, often in spite of inner objections.

Student participation in the development of the Individual Educational Plan is extremely useful when appropriately handled. A student who is old enough or otherwise capable of comprehending and contributing to the discussion can add significant feedback to the thinking of the Committee. Furthermore, participation and commitment to a set of recommendations that are collectively and collaboratively developed increase the chances of success in the form of positive changes in the student's behavior.

The exchange of perspectives and positions at the CSE meeting can be constructive if all sides feel that they offer meaningful feedback, emanating from slightly different vantage points.

School-based service personnel can be instrumental in turning an adversarial situation into a complementary exchange through seeking parents' views and respecting the inner logic with which they handle their problems.

The presence of the out-of-school agency or private therapist at CSE meetings can be instrumental in reducing school-family tensions. He or she can maintain a neutral role as a "third party" or as family advocate. A neutral position enables the therapist to bring to bear communication strategies that help the two parties negotiate their positions. In the role of a "third party," the therapist may help reduce the emotional intensity inherent in the situation. The presence of an advocate may enable the family to feel more powerful and therefore less defensive and more open to constructive problem solving. The therapist, knowing the child and the family, can encourage their participation and add his or her own input into the decision-making process.

e. Phase II of the Individual Educational Plan and Follow-up

The second phase of the IEP development (IEP–Phase II) consists of setting short-range instructional goals, methods for their attainment, and criteria for evaluation of progress. Although this endeavor is carried out primarily by the classroom teacher, the parent is given an opportunity to join in the process, make suggestions, and offer relevant information.

Progress of students in special education is subject to an annual review and a triannual full evaluation. Participation by the family and the out-of-school practitioner is again crucial at this junction. Changes occurring at home may be as important to consider as those emerging at school. Differences between the school and the family may appear again. Although a teacher may recommend continuation of the program, the parents and therapist may emphasize the benefits inherent in a program that offers more independence and less supportive services. The school may recommend gradual termination of special programs, while the family may be eager to see total "graduation" or full continuation in the special program.

A total progress assessment that takes into account changes at school and at home as well as the student's feeling about the program will undoubtedly result in greater accuracy and better prediction of future success. The therapist is again instrumental at this point in helping both sides consider the total picture and making useful recommendations based on an intimate knowledge of the child and the family.

f. The Special Education Model and Other School Services

The referral-evaluation-intervention–follow-up process outlined above offers an excellent model for service provision and school-family collaboration in less formally structured mental health school programs. The central goal of enhancing school-family-student collaboration can be served well by utilizing a variety of systems models to be described in detail in Chapters 3 and 4.

III. THE BUILDING ADMINISTRATION SUBSYSTEM

Relationship patterns between school building administrators, school service personnel, classroom teachers, students, and parents follow interactional patterns similar to those adhered to by families and other social organizations.

1. Hierarchy. School administrators stand in a clearly higher hierarchical position to staff in terms of power, leadership, and authority. Variations exist, however, in the nature of boundaries between the hierarchies. Boundaries may be rigid, loose and blurred, or clear and flexible.

When rigid boundaries prevail, the school tends to be run as a "tight ship." Principals instruct teachers, who further instruct their students in a similar manner. Memoranda and announcements are the usual mode of communication. Participation in decision making and program development by teachers is minimal. Similarly, parents' and teachers' feedback and participation is rarely sought. This is an administration high on structure and efficiency but low on exchange and collaboration.

Loose and blurred boundaries between administration and staff are often a source of confusion which, at times, borders on chaos. Rules are ambiguous and inconsistently enforced. Teachers are left to their own devices and are poorly supervised. A sense of anxiety and abandonment felt by teachers often spills over to students.

Clear and flexible boundaries retain the hierarchical structure but provide for frequent communication, sharing, and collaboration between staff and administration. This style often serves as a model for the classroom style of interaction. It also offers a fertile ground for exchange between families and the school administration.

A school administrator increases his or her ability to enhance collaborative modes of interaction by using systems relationship principles and techniques. The following are a few examples:

2. Triadic interactions. Administrators often find themselves involved in a variety of triangular relationships: parent-teacher-principal triangle; teacher-student-principal triangle; teacher-service-staff-principal triangle; and so on. A parent-teacher-principal triangle may surface when a principal has to take a position with regard to conflicting demands or opinions of parent and teacher. Such differences may appear on issues of placement (special programs, retention), homework, discipline, and many others. On one hand, a principal may be committed to supporting the teacher. On the other, he or she may wish to be open to parents and consider their position very earnestly.

A teacher-student-principal triangle often develops when situations such as these take place: A student complains to the principal about a teacher; a teacher demands more severe disciplinary action than deemed necessary by the principal; a student requests a change of teacher assignment; or a teacher requests removal of a student from his or her class. Conflicts of this nature are among the most common situations calling for a resolution of triadic interactions.

Conflicting pulls among various staff members, staff and families, students and teachers are inevitable and are well known to any administrator. They resolve such issues in various ways: advocating one of the opposing views, compromising, referring issues to committees, and meeting with the opposing parties to help them find a common ground. The latter seems to come closest to the approach used by therapists in helping to resolve conflicts. Such an attitude enables the administrator to avoid being caught in a one-sided alliance. Seeing a student's needs from the perspective of different subsystems within the organization can help achieve a relative detriangulated position most conducive to problem solving.

Therapists can be instrumental in assisting school organizations adopt a systemic approach. They can model system intervention techniques when they act as consultants either for individual students or for programs. Consultation services to schools will be described in greater detail in Chapter 5.

IV. GOVERNMENT, CENTRAL ADMINISTRATION, AND THE FAMILY THERAPIST

Therapists have little opportunity to interact directly with the other subsystem involved in forming school policy. As a group, however, therapists have an obligation to take a position and attempt to influence legislators on a number of issues affecting children and their families. Through lobbying, publishing, and participation in national conferences as well as local and national committees therapists need to address a number of crucial issues affecting families, such as:

1. Day care and free preschool education guaranteed;
2. Maternal and paternal leave of absence during early infancy;
3. Elimination of classification labels as a condition for eligibility to special education services;
4. Amend welfare programs to promote intactness of families; and
5. Support for inclusion of mental health and family therapy services in government subsidized medical plans.

On a central administration level of local school systems, therapists need to address, support, and participate in programs such as:

1. Ongoing staff development programs in family dynamics;
2. Changing gender distribution of classroom and administrative leadership positions;
3. Developing comprehensive school curricula in the area of family relations, sex education, and parenting;
4. Assisting teenage mothers who remain in school in obtaining parenting skills; and
5. Developing a coherent policy with regard to parent participation in school affairs.

Therapists are in a position to assist in the development of these goals and many others as consultants and trainers on the school buildings or school district levels, as well as in other systems such as the courts, the church, gangs, and Little League.

V. CONCLUSION

The central goal of enhancing school-family collaboration can be well served and perpetuated by utilizing a variety of system-based models. Some of these models will be discussed in Chapters 3 and 4. A variety of informal consultation strategies will be discussed in Chapters 5, 6, and 7.

At this point, however, it might be helpful to keep in focus a number of systemic principles as they apply to school-family collaboration.

Students and homes can be viewed as one large system in which all participants—teachers, administrators, support personnel, students, parents, and extended families—are active participants. A student's symptomatic behavior is therefore seen in the context of the total interactive system rather than just as a function of an "internal" problem, a home problem, or a school problem alone.

Schools and families are seen as subsystems that work in synchrony or run into conflict at different times. Children often function as a third party in a dynamic triangle. There are no "victims" or "villains" in the large school-family system but rather different parts of the system affecting one another. The mental health practitioner, whether entering the system or remaining outside, is instrumental in enhancing communication and empowering its participants.

A number of models for school-family-therapist collaboration have been developed. The next few chapters will offer examples of such models.

CHAPTER 3

EXAMPLES OF COLLABORATIVE CONSULTATION MODELS

This chapter will summarize and discuss five theoretical models described in the literature that have applicability for the private therapy practitioner who is interested in working directly with the school system in conjunction with individual and family treatment. These are the Ackerman Family Institute's School Collaboration Model (Weiss & Edwards, 1992), an Adlerian Consultation Model (Nicoll, Platt, & Platt, 1983), the Ecosystemic Treatment Model (Lusterman, 1992), the Family Systems Intervention Model (Beal & Chertkov, 1992), and the Crisis Intervention Model (Steele and Raider, 1991).

As described earlier, it is important to see the school as a system. It is also necessary to note that the family, too, operates as a system. A solar system, a judicial system, an electrical system, a banking system, and a family system, to name a few, all have one thing in common: interacting components, units, or subsystems influencing and being influenced by each other. Goldenberg and Goldenberg (1991) define families as "living, ongoing entities, organized wholes with members in a continuous, interactive patterned relationship with one another extending over time and space" (p. 33). There are a number of other sources as well that describe the concept of the family as a system (Boyd-Franklin, 1989; Carter & McGoldrick, 1988; Gurman & Kniskern, 1991; Hoffman, 1981; Levant, 1984; Minuchin & Fishman, 1981). In addition, key family therapy concepts, including those of boundaries and joining (Sherman, Oresky, & Rountree, 1991), complementarity, enactment, and reframing (Minuchin & Fishman, 1981), and so on, have been elaborated on elsewhere.

Lightfoot (1978) points out that because of different perceptions and expectations of each other and of the children, families and schools are frequently in conflict. The desirability for parents and schools to function as partners is underscored by Carl and Jurkovic (1983), who cite some of the problems that can arise when therapists working with children do not have direct access to school personnel. They point out that often the problems that children exhibit at school do not surface at home. Also, information from the school to the parents can become distorted when the parents attempt to communicate it to the therapist. In addition, without the interface between school, parents, and therapist, cross blaming might well occur. Woody, Yeager, and Woody (1990) believe family therapy to be important in making school-based decisions for handicapped children, noting that Federal legislation actually mandates family involvement. They argue that although a school professional might introduce family issues, having an outside family therapy consultant avoids any suspicions of conflict of interest, allays fears of subjectivity, and ensures having a person with a high level of clinical training and, even possibly, experience in negotiation and mediation.

Finally, children's behavior patterns develop within and are shaped by the family. The power of family systems to be either supportive or sabotaging influences on the behavior and/or academic achievement of their members is well documented (Golden, 1984; Nicoll, 1984). What follow are family-school consultation models that reflect an appreciation for and an integration of family systems theory in the collaboration between private practitioner and school in working with children with emotional, behavioral, and/or academic problems.

I. THE ACKERMAN FAMILY INSTITUTE'S SCHOOL COLLABORATION MODEL

A. Theoretical Considerations

Weiss and Edwards (1992) explain that their family-school collaboration model is founded on two important sets of concepts: Tagiuri's (1968) work on organizational climates and Seeman's (1968) notions of social connectedness.

There are four elements that Tagiuri identifies as impacting upon a school's climate or internal environment and thus affecting how those involved with the school relate to it and to each other. The first element is the school's ecology. This takes into account not only the quality and quantity of the physical space and resources, such as equipment, furnishings, and educational materials, but also includes the characteristics and resources of the community. The second element is the school's milieu or personal demographics. This entails a close examination of such things as the students' ethnic and cultural background, level of motivation, and educational and vocational achievement and experiences. The third element is the social system or relationship patterns that exist among the school staff, students, and family members. The fourth element is the culture of the school system, which encompasses the beliefs, values, and expectations of all involved.

These elements enable one to examine ways in which the school either promotes or prohibits a collaborative atmosphere between families and the school. The ideal situation is a shared "school culture," that is, where the school personnel and the students and their families hold similar beliefs, values, and meanings. Where that does not already exist, a close examination of the above elements permits the modifications necessary to bring about more collaboration and sharing.

The set of concepts based on Seeman's (1968) work on social connectedness posits that connectedness or alienation is a function of power, meaning, norms, inclusion, and self-relatedness. Weiss and Edwards (1992) discuss each of these concepts. Parents who have a sense of power and expect that their actions can have a positive impact on their children's school performance are more likely to share in the school's efforts to help their children succeed. The concept of meaning refers to the idea that relevant information must be consistently shared between schools and families. For example, changes at home for the student may clarify for teachers the meaning of any behavioral changes in the student. Only when there is sufficient information can future predictions and appropriate decisions be made. Cooperation increases when parents understand the norms of the school, that is, how they are expected to interact with the school and be of greatest help in assisting their children within the school system.

The degree to which families feel included in the school system depends to a great extent on cultural differences and shared values. Through a sharing of ideas about school expectations, school personnel and families can cooperatively develop common educational goals for the children. The concept of self-relatedness refers to the intrinsic pleasure that can be derived from participating in an activity because of the good that it does rather than merely to avoid being "blamed" for something. For example, to help a child master mathematics should be perceived as valuable and rewarding rather than as a way to prevent criticism for having a child who is deficient in that area.

True collaboration in a school exists when concepts such as openness, connectedness, cooperation, and respect are part of the experiences of staff, students, and family alike (Weiss & Edwards, 1992).

B. The Model

The focus of this model is for private practitioner consultants to train school teams to work collaboratively with parents and children. The Ackerman Project was developed in 1981 and has involved over 50 New York City schools. Weiss and Edwards (1992) identify three major obstacles to the formation of collaboration between families and schools. First, there are usually no established ongoing procedures for problem solving and information sharing between the school and the family. Second, cultural, racial, and economic differences between school personnel and families often create difficulties in effective communication. Third, parents are seldom viewed as "partners or co-decision-makers" by the school. The task of the consultant in this model is to provide the training program to enable the families and schools to overcome these barriers.

In this model the independent practitioner, as consultant, also becomes an example by forming a collaborative relationship in his or her interactions with school personnel. According to Weiss and Edwards (1992), after two to three years very little, if any, consultant support will be necessary. At that point the program will have been incorporated into the staff's daily routine.

1. Prerequisites for Success

The first prerequisite is that of commitment on the part of the school administration. The school principal must not only sincerely believe in the concept of school-family collaboration, but also must convey his or her commitment to all of the school personnel, students, and parents at every opportunity.

In addition, there should be a coordinating committee consisting of the principal, school psychologist, social worker, and guidance counselor with representation from teachers and parents. This committee assesses the current family-school relationship, identifies areas of need, and keeps the rest of the school and parents informed. Such a structure has been found to increase ownership of the process and to facilitate greater involvement by all concerned.

Another prerequisite is to have someone in the school be family-school coordinator with responsibility for initiating, organizing, and facilitating activities that will improve family-school relationships. That person can be any professional, including school psychologist, assistant principal, guidance counselor, or social worker.

2. *Interventions*

After the needs of the group requesting assistance are taken into account, a decision must be made whether to train the entire staff or to train a small team. Experience has led Weiss and Edwards (1992) to determine that when a small team of educators and parents are trained and they then take responsibility for disseminating what they have learned to the rest of the school, there is greater staff ownership of the process.

Team training is especially effective when there is a districtwide initiative aimed at family-school collaboration, as teams from several schools can be trained simultaneously and they have the added benefit of learning from each other. In addition to the team training, there are consultations, demonstrations, and workshops. According to Weiss and Edwards (1992) it takes two to three years for significant change in the school climate to occur.

a. Training sessions. These provide a conceptual framework and the specific techniques that participants will use when they collaborate with families. Weiss and Edwards list seven content areas that include viewing the family and school as belonging to one system; looking at ways to support students' educational goals; acquiring strategies to change alienated and adversarial family-school relationships to collaborative ones; interviewing techniques and follow-up procedures. This training is done through lectures, offering examples and providing learning exercises such as role plays, simulated family-school meetings, "blame-blocking" exercises, and the showing of videotapes.

b. Consultation sessions. These allow the school staff to have active participation in the planning and implementation of activities, which are geared to help them obtain their goals.

The process includes defining the staff's concerns, priorities, intervention targets, specific goals, and actual activity, including a follow-up.

c. Modeling collaboration. The examples shown by the consultant in the course of leading family-school meetings provide positive experiential feedback for the school staff, parents, and students. They see new approaches to dealing with different problems that can, in turn, lead to new attitudes.

II. AN ADLERIAN CONSULTATION MODEL

A. Theoretical Considerations

A basic tenet of Adlerian theory is that all continuing behavior is purposeful, goal-directed, and socially understandable. Because the family is seen as being in perpetual movement, the therapist's task becomes one of identifying, interpreting, and redirecting what is being dysfunctionally reenacted constantly (Dinkmeyer & Sherman, 1989). Thus, collaboration between the therapist and the school provides a natural setting in which the therapist can explore, compare, and understand the child's behavior not only from the vantage point of what occurs in the therapist's office setting but also in contrast to how that behavior shows up or fails to show up in the school and what the behavior means in both contexts.

Another task of Adlerian family therapy is to help families understand the goals they set for themselves, as their behaviors are directed by their striving to attain these goals. The goals are evolved from beliefs, myths, and lifestyles. Some goals are fictional in that they represent unrealistic or faulty views, such as "If I am perfect everyone will love me." Identifying and exploring faulty assumptions will help the family to become more cooperative and unified in their quest toward more constructive rather than mistaken goals (Dinkmeyer & Sherman, 1989).

B. The Model

Nicoll, Platt, and Platt (1983) justify providing parent-teacher education and family counseling services in the school as an economical way to provide counseling to all families who need it. Widespread access to counseling services does not appear to be available. Although school counselors and psychologists are being called upon more and more frequently to provide counseling (Nicoll, 1984; O'Brien, 1976; Williams, Robinson, & Smaby, 1988), the reality is that they seldom have either the time or the training to do so.

Although school-based family counseling might be viewed by some families as a less threatening source of treatment than seeing an independent practitioner or visiting a counseling agency or clinic, there are certainly a number of families that would feel more comfortable having some separation between their child's school and the family's treatment. In any case, the practitioner can function as a link or bridge between school and family in those situations where private counseling is sought outside the school either because of necessity or preference.

In the Adlerian model the therapist provides psychoeducation through lectures on such issues as child rearing and development. The practitioner with a sound understanding of family dynamics and child behavior can also serve as facilitator in parent-teacher conferences, which seek to explore the student's problem behavior and to offer teachers effective interventions to deal with the problem. With her schedule flexibility and expertise in human relations, the therapist is likely to be highly sought after and thought of as a resource both within and outside of the school.

Nicoll, Platt, and Platt (1983) describe the Adlerian family-school conference model as a four-step process. First, the practitioner fosters an atmosphere of openness, sincerity, and honesty. All participants are heard, their views are respected, and they are allowed to disagree. Their feelings are acknowledged and what each thinks would be better is elicited. At this point, understanding, rather than winning, is the goal.

struggles can be avoided with the suggestion that they try to work things out for a period of time and reconvene another conference a few weeks later to determine how things stand. Often some change does take place in the interim.

The fourth step evaluates the outcome of the conference session. Usually parents and school staff are pleased with the outcome of such conferences and are not only receptive to future collaborative efforts but are also likely to share their experience with other colleagues, which can lead to referrals for the therapist.

An extension of facilitating parent-teacher education programs might be for the private practitioner to function as a consultant to the teacher in the classroom, helping him or her to understand and adopt Adlerian techniques, such as the class meeting, the use of metaphors, and interpersonal relationship training, including conflict resolution (Nicoll, Platt, & Platt, 1983).

III. THE ECOSYSTEMIC TREATMENT MODEL

A. Theoretical Considerations

Lusterman (1992) describes an ecosystemic approach as one that considers the interaction of two or more subsystems. In the case of a dysfunctional child, the two main subsystems involved are the family and the school. An ecosystemic intervention is integrative as well as sequential. It is integrative in that the intervention accommodates various theoretical positions such as individual and family systems therapies. And it is sequential as it continuously assesses a problem and prescribes solutions until the particular issue has been satisfactorily resolved, what Lusterman calls "describing, prescribing, and redescribing." He posits that the ecosystemic approach fosters outreach and a collaboration between many elements of the ecosystem. This makes the therapist more aware of her own role within the system and, in addition, provides her with an opportunity to receive feedback from peers and to foster greater accountability for the private practitioner, who often functions somewhat in an atmosphere of professional isolation.

B. The Model

Lusterman (1992) suggests Olson's (1986) Circumplex Model as a formal way to evaluate the family's level of functioning. The evaluation system for the family looks at three variables: the degree of closeness in a family, its ability to change, and the effectiveness of its communications. Lusterman has adapted Olsen's Clinical Rating Scale so that it may be used by the clinician to evaluate how the school team is structured and how it communicates both internally and with the family. It is only after the evaluation process that significant strategies and appropriate interventions can be made.

1. Evaluating the School-Family Relationship

Although one can get a sense of how the school team works and how members of that team relate to the parents and child by asking the family to describe its interactions, a more accurate picture might be drawn from the therapist's having direct contact with the school. The therapist should inform parents that therapy is most effective when she can freely contact the school and that her usefulness is lessened when that is not possible. Although some families might be reluctant to give such permission, they usually do so once trust is established (Lusterman, 1992).

Carefully listening to how the guidance counselor, social worker, school psychologist, nurse, teacher, and administrator convey the problem allows the therapist to form some immediate hypotheses regarding the school team's opinion of the family, whether they are affixing blame or offering support and if they see the school as contributing to the problems in any way. The therapist will want to learn of individual teachers' attitudes about the child as well as any instances of interactions between the child and other school personnel. Sometimes the child and his or her problem are viewed quite differently by various people in the school, and that situation could well contribute to the problem the child is experiencing. Lusterman (1991) notes that the school seldom sees itself as part of the problem in much the same way as parents usually do not consider themselves to be part of the problem when their child is experiencing difficulties. He suggests that, again, the avoidance of blame and the attitude of collegial sharing of information and ideas will allow for a good working relationship between the consultant and the school.

2. Modulating the School-Family Relationship

Occasionally the therapist must recommend that direct contact between the family and the school cease for a specified period of time. During this period the school and the family agree that all school contacts be made to the therapist. This intervention usually occurs when a school bombards an enmeshed and chaotic family with negative reports about the child. The family often become even more disorganized and unable to effectively manage the child whose behavior, in turn, worsens. Such a recommendation from the therapist can also be made when an adversarial relationship has built up between the family and the school or when a deep split among the school personnel has rendered it impossible to clearly negotiate or communicate with the family. In this event, the therapist clarifies what are home as opposed to school problems and also helps define the responsibilities of the child, the school, and the family for themselves and to each other.

The therapist works with the school on school-related issues and with the family on nonschool-related problems. As the problems begin to ease, the therapist, serving as a catalyst, fosters a gradual reinvolvement of the school and parental systems.

Just as disengagement between the school and the family can be needed, sometimes the therapist must help the school and family become more engaged. This can become necessary when the school is poorly organized and lax, or if the family is emotionally unavailable, lacks sufficient parental control, or both. Here the therapist must find a way to mobilize both the school and the family to provide appropriate supervision and limit setting. Sometimes other agencies must be brought in to help the school and family, such as family court or a parent support group.

Any progress in the child frequently leads to some sense of success and empowerment and more involvement by the parents. In either case, whether less involvement or more is called for, as the family and school are able to work together more appropriately, the therapist can begin to withdraw.

C. Other Issues

1. Confidentiality

Ecosystemic therapy poses some complicated issues about confidentiality. Individual family members, the family as a whole, or the school might request that certain information not be shared and that secrets be maintained. Aside from the legal injunctions against confidentiality, such as in cases of abuse or life-threatening situations, Lusterman (1991) reports that he will hold in confidence anything the person revealing the information does not want to share. He states that in his experience the person who has requested confidentiality usually spontaneously shares it at a later date. What he considers most important is that the confidentiality limits be clearly outlined to all concerned at the beginning of therapy and that those rules be strictly maintained. Only then can the ecosystem have confidence in the therapist's role.

2. Telephone Consultation

Lusterman (1992) sees telephone consultations with members of the school team to be an inexpensive yet fast and effective way of intervening. He sets up a "hotline" with the school, a special number where he can be reached at any time during the day, including the times when he is in session. In his experience, responding briefly to school personnel during sessions is accepted by the family whose session is interrupted, often presenting for that family a model of how problems can be resolved. It is also seen as evidence of the need for open communication. Of course the identity of the family being discussed is kept confidential, and when more time is needed, appropriate arrangements are made for such calls. These telephone consultations can be used to help teachers assess and modify their approach to a student, to resolve issues in the school system itself, and even to allow more informal approaches to problems that might otherwise be met with defensiveness on the part of school personnel.

3. Impartiality

Although the independent practitioner is hired by the family, Lusterman (1991) believes that the therapist's task is one of facilitating change rather than one of being an advocate. This stance permits the therapist to join with different members of the ecosystem at various times depending upon what is taking place in the therapy.

IV. A FAMILY SYSTEMS MODEL

A. Theoretical Considerations

Beal and Chertkov (1992) use Murray Bowen's family systems theory as the foundation for their perspective. They posit that two forces influence human growth and development. One is individuality and autonomy and the other is togetherness and fusion. The balance between the two can be seen not only in the way family members relate to one another but also in the relationship between family and school.

The degree of differentiation or individuality determines how well families respond to stress, with the more highly differentiated family generally being well-defined, better able to adapt, and less likely to develop symptoms. This also holds true for the child and parent faced with a school-related problem. The greater the autonomy, the more likely the child can appropriately cope with whatever problem arises.

Beal and Chertkov (1992) state that chronic stress within a family generally leads to one of four complaints. There are problems of marital conflict, emotional or physical distancing, a dysfunctional spouse, or child-focused problems. Parental emotional focus on a child as a means of dealing with family stress can lead to that child becoming vulnerable to a number of symptoms, including school difficulties.

The family systems perspective conceptualizes such symptoms as distortions or imbalances in family relationships. Therefore, therapy must consider the entire family unit when attempting to modify its relationships and symptoms.

B. The Model

The therapist must first identify relationship patterns and discover the role that the symptoms play within the family's emotional system. This is most effectively accomplished by not only observing interactions within the family but also the relationship between the family and the school system. Meetings with the entire family and with all involved school personnel both separately and in combination are needed to make the appropriate observations.

Next, the therapist must ascertain each family member's part in setting up and maintaining the pattern. This entails looking at the family hierarchy; examining the boundaries within each system and subsystem as well as between systems; considering alliances and coalitions; judging the members' functioning capacities; and evaluating what meaning system members place on the child's problem behavior (Carlson, 1992).

Then the therapist attempts to shift the emotional focus from the child to the marital relationship. This must be done slowly, especially in highly intense families with a strong need to see that all the problems are within the child. To move too quickly with such families is to risk their prematurely leaving therapy. The therapist helps the parents examine the child's school difficulties and intervenes with the school to clarify its expectations of the child and to identify appropriate educational resources if they are necessary. The role of reduction of anxiety in the system as a way of addressing the child's symptoms is important. Collaboration with the school may serve to reduce such anxiety.

V. THE CRISIS INTERVENTION MODEL

A. Theoretical Considerations

Steele and Raider (1991) define families in crisis as those who have been unable to successfully cope with changes that have taken place within their family system. They add that it is not the event per se but rather the perception of that event as being overwhelming, dangerous, or uncontrollable that defines it as a crisis. Therefore, two families can experience the same situation but react quite differently.

Families unable to resolve perceived threats often move into a state of crisis, and in an effort to rid themselves of the fear and anxiety, they embrace self-defeating behavior such as avoidance, denial, substance abuse, and so on. Crisis intervention with families in the schools can serve to replace self-defeating behaviors with effective and adaptive methods to successfully manage the anxiety as well as the crisis.

The crisis method is appropriate within the school setting because a crisis is time-limited, usually lasting no more than a few weeks (Steele & Raider, 1991). The need for help is immediate. Steele and Raider refer to "limited community resources, long waiting lists, and the reluctance of families to engage in treatment..." (p. 14) as reasons why crisis intervention in the school can be effective. Also during the crisis the family is experiencing pain, which makes them more amenable to interventions seen as a means of alleviating the distress. Finally, the problem-solving approach used in crisis intervention is within the boundaries of the school's responsibility to provide guidance, support, and stabilization through learning new skills, both for students and their families.

B. The Model

This is a 12-stage model that is to be completed within the first interview but not necessarily in the order presented here. The focus of sessions held subsequently will depend upon the individual family and the nature of the crisis.

1. Along with attempting to minimize increased anxiety and to prevent further family deterioration, this stage establishes ground rules for intervention. It apprises the family about what it can expect, what it can do to help and what the alternatives are if the intervention does not work. This allows the family to give its informed consent and commitment and to gain some sense of control.
2. The family is helped to understand the crisis through identifying any possible distortions surrounding the causes and threats of the crisis.
3. The therapist must clearly examine her perception of the crisis and determine if it is similar to the family's, and if it is not, be aware of what the differences are so that the process is focused and clear.
4. The specific nature of the family system must be understood to ensure that appropriate and useful interventions are made.
5. Boundaries, subsystems, strengths, and barriers to a healthy resolution of the crisis must be identified.
6. The level of danger for the family to engage in danger-

ous and/or self-destructive behavior must be assessed. If the potential for such behavior exists, safeguards must be established immediately.

7. This stage involves normalizing the family's responses to the crisis and providing some hope that the crisis can be stabilized, resolved, or managed. When families are in crisis, knowing that their reactions are to be expected in such situations and that their reactions are not unlike those of others in similar situations can alleviate anxiety. The family realizes it is not abnormal and can feel that the therapist has had experience working with similar problems.

8. The means of minimizing destructive and/or self-defeating expressions of feelings are explored. More positive expressions are sought and energy is channeled into activities aimed at resolving the crisis while preserving relationships.

9. The family is helped to feel empowered through learning problem-solving skills to deal not only with the current crisis but also with any crisis that might arise in the future.

10. The family is taught how to identify solutions and through that process experiences a sense of ownership in its treatment and increased confidence.

11. The family should be helped to arrive at a solution in the therapist's office that is practical. This should occur before they leave that first session. Role playing is an effective way for the family to rehearse its chosen solution, as it is a technique that builds confidence and decreases anxiety.

12. This last stage involves a reassessing of the family's status. It provides the therapist an opportunity to check with the family to determine if they feel more hopeful and more in control. It also permits the family to receive additional support and a referral for longer-term help if that is appropriate. It is important to remember that in crisis intervention the therapist's goal is to return the family to its level of functioning

prior to the crisis rather than to attempt more sweeping changes.

VI. DISCUSSION OF THE COLLABORATIVE CONSULTATION MODELS

The basic premise that supports all five models is the absolute necessity for a working relationship to exist between school personnel and the student and his family. The next shared fundamental is that such collaboration is extremely difficult, if not impossible, to achieve in most instances without a concerted effort on the part of all involved. Everyone agrees it is absolutely vital to optimal success for the student. However, as Weiss and Edwards (1992) point out, even after 15 years of definitive research showing the positive effects of parents' involvement on educational achievement and attitudes as well as on improved school attendance, the American educational system has not sufficiently embraced family involvement. And, finally, it is quite clear that any clinician interested in facilitating or in implementing collaboration between families and the school must acquire a thorough knowledge of school systems.

A. Similarities and Differences

There are more similarities than differences between the five models presented in this chapter. In each model the private practitioner becomes the pivotal force in collaborative negotiations with varying intensity and within different time frames. In the case of the Ackerman Family Institute's Model, the practitioner is more likely to be a member of a team rather than working independently. She is also working with school teams for a minimum of two years. On the other hand, Steele and Raider's (1991) Crisis Intervention Model focuses on a much narrower range, involving a student, his individual family and school personnel, as needed, over a brief period of a few weeks. All private practitioners who work with schoolage children have, no doubt, at some point had to contact that student's school while also being in touch with the youngster's family. The other three models fit along a continuum between the Ackerman and the Crisis Models.

In the Ackerman Model the ultimate goal is to train the school team to eventually take over the functions once served by the consultant so that the family-student-school collaboration becomes an integral part of each student's school experience. The other four models are to sensitize both the family and the school to the advantages of working together collaboratively on behalf of a student who is experiencing problems.

In both the Ecosystemic and the Family Systems Models the practitioner often serves not only as a moderator between family and school systems, but also as a mediator serving to disengage those systems when appropriate, working with each system separately. However, the practitioner's primary goal is to obtain as much information from and cooperation between the school and family as possible in order for her to be most effective in working with the family in treatment.

B. Conclusion

These five models are by no means an exhaustive look at what private practitioners can do to foster collaboration between school personnel and families. However, they do offer a wide range of options for ensuring that all possible avenues for obtaining relevant information are pursued in order to help the students and their families. Whether their intent is to influence the outcome for one family or to do so for all families in a particular school, these guidelines can be adapted for many purposes.

CHAPTER 4

EXAMPLES OF SCHOOL-BASED INTERVENTION MODELS

This chapter examines some important school-based intervention services that recognize and include a family component. These include the School Development Program at Yale University's Child Study Center (Comer, 1993, 1988); the Comprehensive Approach to School Success (CASS) Model at Temple University (Wang, 1992); the ASPECTS 27 Model (B. Schwarz & N. Rothberg, personal communication, 1993); the Queens College IS 227Q Model (P. Woods, personal communication, September 2, 1992); the Community Network Model (Gatti & Colman, 1988); and the School Refusal Programs in Japan (Nakane, 1990; Koizumi, 1990; Murase, 1990). These interventions, although not necessarily based on a family therapy theoretical framework, nevertheless recognize, value, and integrate the concept of family involvement and/or treatment.

I. THE SCHOOL DEVELOPMENT PROGRAM

The Comer (1993, 1988) school-based program has been in existence longer than any of the other models described in this chapter. In 1968 Comer and his colleagues at Yale University's Child Study Clinic began their School Development Program at two schools in New Haven. Fueled by the success of this program in two inner city schools, as measured by greatly improved academic performance and decreased truancy and disciplinary problems, it was subsequently implemented in nearly 300 schools around the country.

A. Theoretical Considerations

This program places more emphasis on generating and promoting supportive ties between children, parents, and school than on some of the more usual academic concerns that stress teaching skills and credentials. Comer (1988) notes that many of the ideas that formed the basis of this program emerged from trying to understand the elements that determine which children, especially poor Black minority children, become successful later in life. He realized that parents who instill a sense of confidence in their children and teach them socialization skills enable their children to utilize whatever educational opportunities arise. He speculated that the basic reason poor children outside the mainstream are more likely to fail stems from an inability to successfully "bridge the social and cultural gap between home and school..." (p. 43). He believes that more focus should be placed on interpersonal factors rather than on curricula and instruction, which often proceed as though all children are in the mainstream of society and come to school equally prepared to learn.

Comer and his colleagues refer to "sociocultural misalignment" to describe the failure to appreciate the existence of significant differences in children's levels of preparedness (Comer, 1988). Such misalignment affects the child's academic success in several ways. The child who lacks social skills is less likely to elicit the kind of positive response from the teacher that leads to the establishment of a close bond between the teacher and that student. Also, expectations for the child at home can be vastly different from those the child faces at school. A child who is quiet, unobtrusive, and avoids making his or her needs known may be regarded as a "good" child at home but may be seen as lacking in sufficient assertiveness and initiative at school. Furthermore, the child's language skills, reading habits, and social skills may be acceptable and seen as the norm at home, but can be considered quite inadequate at school.

Comer (1988) notes that although many poor parents feel alienated from and have few expectations of the school, they nevertheless see the school as the only hope they and their children have for a positive future. He points out that the family's attitudes, values, behaviors, and socialization patterns strongly influence elements crucial to a child's academic development. Thus, the School Development Program seeks to foster academic achievement in the children through positive interactions between parents and school staff, a situation which, in turn, permits bonding between the students and the school. At one school, for example, it was noted that nearly every parent (92%) visited the school an average of once a month following the institution of this program.

Of course, any major change in the organization and management of a school requires the approval and support of the community school board and the school superintendent. The track record of this program over the past 25 years could well overcome any objections to its incorporation in the system if well presented. For example, Comer and Haynes (1992), in summarizing the academic effects of the School Development Program in several school districts, showed that in 1986 one Michigan school area made significant gains in both mathematics and reading. Over a four-year period, four grade levels in the Program schools exceeded the gains made by the schoolwide district as a whole. A 1987 assessment of Prince George's County public schools showed that between 1985 and 1987 students in School Development Program schools achieved significantly higher gains on the California Achievement Test than did the district as a whole. Other school areas have shown positive academic results as well.

There have also been significant results in the School Development Program schools when measures of behavior and school adjustment were evaluated (Comer & Haynes, 1992). Such areas as attendance, suspensions, classroom behavior, and participation and attitude toward authority showed positive change. In addition, dimensions such as students' self-concept (Haynes & Comer, 1990) and parents' and teachers' attitudes regarding overall classroom and school climate (Haynes, Comer, & Hamilton-Lee, 1989) tend to show improvement in School Development Program schools as compared to those schools where a School Development Program does not exist.

Finally, there is a seven-hour series of videotapes (Spillane, 1992), *For Children's Sake: The Comer School Development Program*, with an accompanying manual, that has been developed by Comer and his colleagues at the suggestion of and with the assistance of the Rockefeller Foundation. These tapes and manual illustrate how School Development Programs can be implemented within a school district.

Comer (1988) also states that his ideas found theoretical support in the work of Albert Solnit and his colleagues, who posit that educational reformation stems from direct observations and long-term interventions into the schools. Thus, Comer, together with a social worker, a psychologist and a special education teacher, immersed themselves into the workings of those two New Haven, Connecticut, schools to determine how those schools functioned. Out of that process emerged the School Development Program model.

B. The Model

There are nine components to the School Development Program (Comer, 1993). They consist of three "mechanisms" that will be discussed in detail as they are the core of the Program, three "operations," and three "guiding principles."

The mechanisms are the Governance and Management Team, the Mental Health or Support Team and the Parents' Program. Of these three mechanisms, the Governance and

Management Team is most important. It carries out the three operations, which include developing a comprehensive academic and social program and school procedures; designing staff development activities; and conducting periodic assessments of the total program to allow for adjustments and modifications of the Program as needed. It also adheres to the three guiding principles. The first principle concerns the leader of the Governance and Management Team, who is usually, but not always, the school principal. It states that neither can the group "paralyze" the leader nor can the leader use the group as a "rubber stamp." When the leader is someone other than the school principal, the principal must remain closely involved in both the meetings and the facilitation of the program. The second principle calls for decisions by consensus rather than by vote to avoid disruptive issues around who did or did not win. The third principle seeks to avoid assigning blame to the various school teams and groups when attempting to resolve problems.

The Governance and Management Team usually consists of 10 to 12 people led by the school principal or his or her designee. The other members include parents and teachers elected by the Parents' Program, a representative of the Mental Health Team, and a nonprofessional support staff person. In addition, in middle and high schools, there are also student representatives.

> Working collaboratively, the Governance and Management Team gives a school a sense of direction, prioritizes and coordinates activities, provides communication, and most importantly, allows everybody to experience a sense of ownership and stake in the outcome of the program in a building. This motivates desirable behavior among parents, staff and students, and the components of the program become synergistic rather than antagonistic. (Comer, 1993, p. 5)

The Mental Health Team consists of the school psychologist, social worker, speech pathologist, and any other support staff, for example a special education teacher. This team is not just concerned with the behavioral problems that actually occur but also focuses on preventing such problems. The case of each student experiencing behavioral, learning, or emotional difficulties is discussed by the team and assigned to a member of the team. Working as a team rather than as separate entities they can track the student and pick up any problematical behavioral patterns.

An example of how the Mental Health Team helped a student, clarified unusual behavior for a teacher, and affected school procedures was illustrated by Comer (1988). A youngster transferred into one of the schools taking part in the intervention program. Upon entering the classroom for the first time, he kicked the teacher and ran out. The team explained to the school staff how the child's behavior was an outgrowth of his anxiety with strangers and not a manifestation of pathology. This prevented the child from being immediately labeled and then treated as "disturbed." This incident, in turn, led to the development of an orientation program to introduce transfer students and their parents to the school.

Other programs to develop out of the team collaboration included a "Discovery Room" for students who showed no interest in school. This intervention permitted a student to remain with the same teacher for two years, building a sense of trust with an adult, while rediscovering an interest in learning through play.

This team also has a delegate on the Governance and Management Team who serves as consultant on child development and relationship issues and recommends and facilitates needed changes in any school procedures that are detrimental to the staff, students, and parents.

The third mechanism of the School Development Program is the Parents' Group. Frequently consultancy programs, especially those formulated by someone outside the school system, are regarded with suspicion not only by school administrators and staff but also by parents. Parents who protest or complain about this new intervention (or what they might view as interference) can be encouraged to join and share their input and concerns as a way of alleviating their misgivings as well as giving them an opportunity to contribute to the team's knowledge about the students and their needs.

Designating a staff person to serve as liaison between the parents and the school is a useful way to facilitate the parents' involvement. Parents are involved in the Program in several ways. They select representatives to serve on the Governance and Management Team, they are active participants in school events, and they, together with staff, plan and support social and academic activities. These activities can range from bake sales and school suppers to holding book fairs, volunteering in the library, or assisting in the classroom as a paid paraprofessional. The good relationships fostered by the collaboration and social activities permit staff and parents to discuss any student problems that might arise without defensiveness and accusations.

> Participation both in the day-to-day program in the classroom as well as in school governance builds parents' confidence and competence as contributors to, and decision makers in, the school community. Such enhancement of parents' social and academic skills has motivated many to return to school and complete their own high school, and in some cases, college education, improving their employment opportunities. (Comer, 1993, p. 6)

II. THE COMPREHENSIVE APPROACH TO SCHOOLING SUCCESS (CASS) MODEL

This Program is a project of Temple University's Center for Research in Human Development and Education. It was designed in collaboration with the Philadelphia Superintendent of Schools, Dr. Clayton, and with Dr. Comer (Wang, 1992). Built upon Comer's School Development Program, it is an integrative school-based model that seeks to provide and coordinate all of the needs of its students, including not only education but also health, nutrition, and socialization and any other areas where there might be concerns.

A. Theoretical Considerations

This program stresses the importance of providing support for students to prevent rather than to remedy failure. It focuses on families with students who are considered at risk either because of low income or because of special needs as evidenced by emotional or behavioral problems. The goal is to help the school determine how best to mobilize and utilize parents, community, and school resources to provide a holistic and comprehensive program for the students.

Children who have participated in preschool programs like Head Start frequently fail to hold onto all of the early gains that resulted from these enrichment programs. The CASS Project serves as a transitional program between Head Start programs and the first four years of elementary school, that is, kindergarten through third grade, for students from low income families.

In addition to an emphasis on collaboration and a process of transition, there is also a recognition that not all students learn in the same way or at the same pace. Thus provisions are made for those differences through individual and small group teaching within the classroom.

B. The Model

There are four major components of the CASS Project. The first is a school development program involved with the establishment of the Planning and Management and the Mental Health Teams. Much of the planning done by the Planning and Management Team is conducted through a workshop forum during which the school staff look at their communities to see how they can access the families and agencies in those communities. The second is a system of instruction that organizes regular classrooms around the needs of the students, including those with special needs. This might take the form of work stations with small groups or even one-on-one instruction. The third component is a structure for securing organizational and resource supports, and the fourth is the family involvement and community connection program.

While outcome statistics for the CASS Program are incomplete, preliminary data collected thus far and representing a two-year effort are quite positive (Oats, personal communication, January 24, 1994). All three schools that are taking part in the project report higher attendance and fewer discipline problems. The schools have also established "parent rooms" and one has added an on-site health clinic. Hard data including the results of standardized testing should be forthcoming soon.

III. THE ASPECTS 27 MODEL

ASPECTS 27 (an acronym for Adolescent, School, Prevention, Education, Counseling, and Training Services) is a nonprofit school- and community-based, multifaceted program serving children and their families in School District 27 of New York City (ASPECTS 27, 1993). The Program, which has been in existence for over 20 years, has several components. It provides ongoing services to the children and their families of 35 public and nonpublic elementary and middle schools.

A. Theoretical Considerations

ASPECTS 27 takes a holistic and family systems approach in working with children. Children and their behavior are seen not only within the context of their families but also within the school and the larger community environments. One of the major components of ASPECTS 27 is the Counseling Center for Family Development. This Center is a school-based clinical prevention program, and it provides a full range of professional services, free of charge, to district children who are seen as experiencing difficulties. Its multi-dimensional efforts are reflected in the fact that it operates under the auspices of two state agencies (the Office of Alcohol and Substance Abuse Services and the Education Department) and it was developed by ASPECTS and a community school district. The goal of the Center is to assist the children to develop more appropriate coping skills, while simultaneously helping their families improve their familial relationships.

B. The Model

Family therapy from a systems theory orientation is the primary treatment of choice. However, the Center also provides individual and group counseling for children and adolescents, marital therapy, and alcohol and chemical dependency counseling for families. When a child has been identified as one in need of treatment, the child's entire family is required to participate in activities ranging from parent-child workshops and seminars to family therapy.

The Center is staffed by trained counselors and by a large number of graduate and postgraduate clinical interns from area colleges and universities. The interns must be either Master's level or post-Master's Certificate level students currently enrolled in a marriage and family therapy or school counseling program or schools of social work. The interns, who receive ongoing clinical training and supervision by program supervisors, are required to commit to a minimum of six contact hours a week for at least one year. Thus, the Center also serves as a training ground for beginning family therapy practitioners.

To accommodate the families, most administration, training, and supervision take place during day hours, while the majority of the families are seen, by appointment, from late afternoon until late evening.

The children are referred by school administrators, guidance counselors, and substance abuse prevention counselors. Families within the district can also self refer. Once the referral is made, the family receives an appointment for a consultation to determine its specific needs.

Other specialized components of ASPECTS 27 include a Summer Program that takes place at day camps and includes student rap and discussion sessions; the coordination of a joint venture with the city police department and the board of education in which police officers conduct workshops on drug abuse for all district fifth and sixth graders; a program with assistant district attorneys to provide a wide variety of services, such as career education and social studies, field trips to learn about the court system, and so on; and Parent Programs in the form of time-limited communication skills workshops covering topics such as parent-child communication, problem-solving skills, and drug awareness and prevention.

When viewed in its entirety, this Model would seem to be a massive undertaking; however, some of the separate components are not only manageable but are relatively easy entrees into a collaborative relationship with any school. For example, a private practitioner might offer a three- or four-week communication skills workshop in a school which provides a needed service to all and allows the administrators, staff, and parents to learn of the practitioner's expertise and availability as a therapist.

IV. QUEENS COLLEGE IS 227Q MODEL

This program represents a 10-year collaboration between a large urban college and a public middle school containing grades five through eight. It was, in part, supported through various grants from the state education department, the U.S. Department of Education, and private foundations, as well as through the support of the faculty and administrators in the College's School of Education. In addition, over 100 interns from the College participated in collaborative projects.

These projects included early morning enrichment classrooms, shows and exhibitions of students' artwork in a school-
community museum; community outreach, and a community
mentorship program which placed eighth graders in voluntary afterschool work sites to foster career orientation and
work experience; a dropout prevention program; and a
Family Clinic where counseling and parent workshops
could be conducted.

A. Theoretical Considerations

The partnership between Queens College and IS 227 was
formulated on the premise that strengthening the schools
and providing the best education possible is "*everybody's* business" (Pflaum & Longo, 1989). Thus college professors,
school teachers and administrators, college graduate interns,
students, and their families worked together on committees
to plan both educational and social activities as well as to
develop proposals for outside funding to support innovative
programs.

Because of this philosophy of inclusion, the school was
made available to all who might need access. Thus, the school
was open two evenings a week until 6, two nights until 10,
and on Saturday mornings. This is an important aspect of
the project. All too often although the desirability of family
and community involvement with the schools is lauded, there
are too few practical provisions made, such as evening hours,
to ensure full participation.

B. The Model

In keeping with the premise that the school should attempt
to meet as many of the students' needs as practical, a Family
Clinic was started by Sidney Trubowitz (P. Woods, personal
communication, September 2, 1992). Students who exhibited behavioral problems or academic difficulties were referred by teachers to a school guidance counselor. The

counselor interviewed the student and then contacted his or her family. If there appeared to be problematical family issues, the counselor would indicate to the families that there were counseling services available through Queens College and that the services were free. The free service meant that every student and his or her family could avail themselves of family treatment.

If the family was amenable to the idea of treatment, the guidance counselor would refer them to the Family Clinic. The director of the Clinic would then match the family to a Queens College student from the Marriage and Family Therapy Program. There were eight such interns a year, and each intern worked with four or five families. In conjunction with conducting family therapy sessions, the interns also consulted with the students' teachers throughout the duration of treatment. The amount of collaboration depended on the needs of the individual students. The families would be seen in counseling through the academic year and, if need be, on a maintenance basis throughout the Summer months as well.

In addition to the family counseling, there were Saturday workshops on topics such as single parenthood and substance abuse. These workshops not only provided family members much needed information, but also generated self-referrals from those who attended them.

The eight interns each received an annual stipend of $1,500 for an eight-hour week. Most internships were for a one-year period, although a few interns served for two years. They received both individual and group supervision. Their training and supervision was provided by Queens College teaching staff. It consisted of didactic course work. The theoretical orientation was based on systems theory. There were also practica and seminars during which the students' cases could be discussed, and they had an opportunity to role play interventions and practice techniques. Each student also presented at a formal case conference and prepared monthly process recordings of his or her counseling sessions.

Because the majority of the interns served for only one year, most of the work with families was short-term counseling, that is, fewer than 15 sessions. Although there are no extensive outcome studies on the efficacy of the treatment, preliminary data based on responses to a questionnaire distributed to several families that participated in the Family Clinic indicate that the families who responded felt the interventions had been helpful (E. Black, personal communication, August 29, 1990).

V. THE COMMUNITY NETWORK MODEL

A. Theoretical Considerations

Gatti and Colman (1988) developed a Community Network Model of collaboration between themselves, as family therapists, the elementary and middle schools of their community, and families with children who were identified as having behavioral problems. Their network model grew out of consultation work in a rather homogeneous community in a small town. The therapists' familiarity with both the schools and the community facilitated their ability to help families secure needed support and services.

Gatti and Colman (1988) use traditional structural family therapy and are guided by four basic principles. The first principle is that the whole family needs to be totally involved in the treatment. The second is that it is important for therapists to be in contact with the significant persons and agencies in the family's life in order to obtain and share relevant information. This might include extended family members, neighbors, social welfare agencies, schools, religious organizations, and social groups as well as other professionals such as physicians. Gatti and Colman note that one must be careful to share information in such a way that boundaries are not violated and harmful psychological labeling is avoided. They add, "Concreteness of style, a focus on systems rather than on individuals, and our constant availability in the network for receiving feedback and modifying our own behavior all help to maintain a sense of the appropriate limits in any given situation" (p. 137).

The third principle is that the child's behavior needs to be interpreted to others in a way that it can be understood even when it cannot be condoned. To this end they avoid psychological jargon and share clear, concrete observations to explain the behavior. An example might be a child whose mother has recently left him in the care of a grandparent and who has begun striking out at other children. School personnel could easily understand this behavior as his taking his anger and frustration out on others and might be more patient and cooperative in working with the therapist as he or she attempts to help the youngster deal with this loss and modify inappropriate behavior.

The last principle is that problems in living should be viewed within a cultural context to reduce guilt and to promote choice. Social mores and rules change rapidly. They find this cultural awareness most salient when there are concerns in the areas of social isolation, sexual standards, sex role styles, political and economic issues, and changing authority structures.

B. The Model

The therapists meet weekly, on a rotating basis, at the various schools to consult with the school personnel, including counselors, nurses, and principals. During the two-hour meetings recommendations are made to the staff regarding ways of handling concerns they have about certain children. Where problems are considered serious enough to warrant family therapy, a school counselor visits the child's parents to make such a recommendation. If the parents agree that treatment or evaluation is needed, they are given the option of working with the consulting therapists.

Gatti and Colman (1988) report having seen a few dozen such referred families during a three-year period. The therapist's first meeting is just with the parents, and it takes place in the therapist's office. They believe that to meet initially with just the parents not only emphasizes their authority, but also allows the parents to be more open and to carefully consider if they wish to pursue treatment with the therapist. The second meeting is in the family's home, and all family members are urged to be present. Families are often pleased that the therapist has taken the time and made an effort to come to where they are. Frequently this is much more convenient for families and permits more members to be present. It also allows the therapist to gain a clearer idea of how the family lives. When family members are absent, it is noted as a disappointment, but the therapist does not refuse to work with the family even if certain members refuse to attend. At the end of each meeting a decision is made about who should participate in the next one. Subsequent meetings take place in various settings, such as in parks and restaurants, and include not only different family subsystems but also friends and neighbors on an as-needed basis. Meeting the people who play major roles in the lives of the family members and seeing the family in different settings provide a wealth of information about the family's functioning.

The authors indicate that they have been successful and note that the families who profited most were those of the working class, perhaps because of the inclusion of an advocacy role on the part of the therapists.

VI. THE SCHOOL REFUSAL PROGRAMS (JAPAN)

A. Theoretical Considerations

Nakane (1990) reports that "school refusal" among Japanese students in Japan is a serious educational problem that has been recognized and investigated for over 30 years. Nakane (1990) and Koizumi (1990) present findings from several Japanese researchers that reflect factors in addition to those usually associated with explanations of separation anxiety—such as unrealistic and persistent worry that either harm to or separation from a major attachment figure will occur; clinging; nightmares around separation themes; and somatization on school days, to name a few. They point to cultural and socioeconomic conditions, including population density, financial considerations, domestic stability, child-rearing practices, very high educational standards with their attendant pressures, as well as the widespread practice of bullying in schools throughout Japan.

Children who refuse to attend school are described as progressing from a state of tension so severe that they refuse to go to school. That stage is followed by feelings of shame, guilt, and inadequacy to such an extent that the children become isolated and seclusive. Eventually, they respond to their parents' criticism with aggressivity and physical abuse toward their mothers.

B. The Model

Murase (1990) presents a case of school refusal in which she engaged the child, his parents, and the school in the child's individual treatment. The school's cooperation was enlisted to periodically send notices to the student assuring him that he was welcome to return to school, which he eventually did. In fact, of the 30 school refusal cases listed by Murase, she had contact with nearly two-thirds of the schools. She also suggests that classmates be encouraged to visit the school refuser and that teachers be engaged to accompany the school refuser to school. No information about outcomes was reported.

Although the interventions and expectations reflected in this Japanese model might not appear to be radical to many of us in this country, given some of the cultural differences in Japan, they represent a giant leap. In Japanese culture one should not fail, and if by some misfortune one does fail, it should never be publicly disclosed. Therapists would do well to keep such cultural differences in mind and consider the usefulness of conservative interventions when working with cultures that attach shame and disgrace to public awareness of problematic behavior within the family.

VII. DISCUSSION OF THE SCHOOL-BASED INTERVENTION MODELS

These models range from the rather complex structure of the School Development Program (Comer, 1993), involving several teams of people, to the much simpler School Refusal Programs in Japan (Murase, 1990). Having such a range from which to choose ensures that each practitioner can select the model most suited to his or her needs. Today, the trend toward group practices makes team interventions more feasible than they were in the past, especially when each mental health worker has a particular specialty. On the other hand, Gatti and Colman's networking model is easily managed by an individual practitioner who could cover as many or as few schools as practical for his or her particular practice.

O'Callaghan (1993), in discussing the "politics" of collaboration, suggests that because most educators think intrapsychically rather than systemically or ecosystemically, the consultant who wishes to establish a collaborative relationship in a school often faces an arduous and difficult task. In addition to what he calls intrapsychic thinking, he enumerates several other obstacles to school-based collaboration. These obstacles include a propensity for school teachers to see their job as primarily academically focused, leaving the task of discussing nonacademic issues to the "specialists." He does not suggest that specialization is unnecessary but rather that some teachers have become less involved with the total student. He maintains that since all children must attend school and most parents have no way of evaluating how well a school is performing, schools lack accountability, which is also an obstacle. Another obstacle, according to O'Callaghan, is what he refers to as "the level of insight produced in ecosystemic collaborative discussions and meetings" (p. 156), or what might be characterized as educators' counter-transferential issues. He points out that a targeted family's parent-child or marital conflicts discussed in collaborative meetings can parallel problems in the educators' families and result in defensive or avoidant behavior on the part of those educators. Other obstacles may include proprietary and monopolistic institutions, weak school leadership, or the jealous guarding of one's "turf." Although the lack of money is often cited as a serious obstacle to setting up a collaborative model, he suggests that frequently "it is a pseudo-issue manufactured by those opposed to the collaborative model" (p. 158).

Mention is made of these obstacles not to discourage one from establishing school-based collaboration. They are offered here merely to forewarn the private practitioner, alerting him or her to possible problems that may have to be negotiated. As noted in Chapter 3, some of the models presented require two or three years to become firmly implanted in the school system. O'Callaghan (1993) notes that in his experience it often took an educator one or two years after hearing his presentation to contact him for further discussion.

The descriptions of the various models outlined in this and the previous chapter provide numerous strategies the private practitioner can use in establishing and supporting a collaborative process. O'Callaghan (1993) proposes that the very first task is to identify someone within the school who is interested in the collaborative model and is willing to be a contact person working within the school system to facilitate introductions and presentations. The next steps should be to meet with school district leaders and to start a pilot project using one or more of these models as a guide.

The next three chapters outline our conceptualization of a collaborative consultation model as it is carried out through the referral, assessment, intervention, and follow-up processes.

CHAPTER 5

COLLABORATION IN THE IDENTIFICATION AND REFERRAL PROCESS

Only a portion of children and families who need therapeutic help get referred for therapy. Only a small group of those referred follow up, and of those seeking therapy, fewer remain in therapy long enough to experience lasting change.

There are many obstacles to bringing children and their families into therapy and maintaining their involvement in the process. They include problems in need identification, in attitudes, and in the referral process.

A. THE IDENTIFICATION PROCESS

Children who need therapeutic intervention may be identified in a number of ways. Their problems may be recognized either by the parent, another family member, the pediatrician, the court system, child protective services, or school personnel.

The schools are the only referral agents who have attempted systematic early identification and intervention programs.

Programs mandated by Federal and State laws and regulations have been instrumental in the identification of handicapped children from birth to age 21. These mandates resulted in nationwide educational opportunities for many children who had been previously neglected and ignored. These programs, however, have two main limitations: (1) they are not comprehensive enough to achieve the educational goals they were set up to achieve; and (2) they are not designed to identify the mental health needs of all children at risk.

1. Educational Limitations

School systems throughout the country, some in response to legislative guidelines and some at their own initiative, have constituted screening programs to identify children with potential learning problems. These include testing during kindergarten registration or during first grade. A screening evaluation is sometimes performed when a new student transfers to the school. Such procedures, which are conducive to the development of early intervention practices, are rarely repeated in higher grades. Students who were missed at the primary level may, therefore, fail to be identified until they exhibit major problems. Screening procedures are by definition rather inexact instruments intended to be followed by more precise assessment tools when a problem is identified. Unfortunately, only the most severe and unambiguously identified children are followed by more intensive testing. Borderline students or those who have problems that are not tapped by the particular tests are often missed. There is also a tendency for such procedures to pick up a substantial number of false positives. Children may thus be unnecessarily labeled or given unneeded costly services.

2. Overlooking Mental Health Needs

The most serious limitation of existing screening programs is that they address only a narrow band of students, namely, the educationally impaired. There remains a large group of children who have emotional and social problems that are often neither identified early nor targeted for special services. These include:

- Children alienated from the social system;
- Children involved in substance abuse;
- Homeless children.;
- Children living in foster homes, custodial facilities, or in temporary residence with relatives;
- Teenage parents and their children;
- Children of addicted, alcoholic, or AIDS-infected parents;
- Children experiencing severe loss due to death, incarceration of a parent, divorce, or abandonment; and
- Children living in economic poverty or subject to severe economic fluctuations in the family.

These children often get identified only after they manifest severe dysfunctional symptoms. The symptoms may include poor academic achievement, nonconforming behavior, excessive absence or truancy, leaving school, defiance of authority, violence against teachers and peers, substance abuse, and suicide.

Problems such as these are not difficult to identify when they become full fledged. At such a point, however, a problem may not only constitute a primary handicap, but it also sets the stage for the development of numerous secondary problems that further exacerbate the original problem, making it exceedingly difficult to either arrest or reverse.

In spite of limited funds and diminishing resources, school systems are making sincere efforts to meet the needs of children in distress. Among the various programs designed to address the needs of at-risk populations are drop-out prevention; substance abuse education and counseling; vocational education; parenting education and counseling; counseling children of divorce; training in violence control and mediation techniques; special educational structures, such as school within schools; and parent and community participation.

Such programs may be successful due to the efforts of talented and devoted educators. However, because of their dependence on financial grants, they are both episodic and subject to premature termination. Furthermore, identification of candidates for such programs often fits the characteristics outlined in the grant requirements rather than the needs of the overall at-risk population.

3. The Role of the Mental Health Practitioner

At present, private practitioners as well as therapists working in agencies have little impact in determining identification policies and procedures. This is due primarily to the separate existence led by the schools and out-of-school practitioners. It is proposed here that the "fenced-in" position of the therapist needs to be changed. Greater involvement in the affairs of local schools and school systems is essential. Although difficulties may exist in penetrating the school's own "fenced-in" establishment, it is possible to do so by employing such strategies as

- Frequent contacting of teachers, pupil services personnel, and administrators in relation to individual cases;
- Volunteering to assist in the development of in-service training programs in early identification;
- Consulting on assessment and program development;
- Participating in the decision-making process of local boards of education by joining such bodies or attending their open meetings; and
- Addressing community groups through adult education and other local associations.

A higher degree of participation may very well increase the flow of referrals from schools to therapists, but more importantly, it helps address the needs of children and helps bring students and their families into treatment.

Mental health agencies can increase their collaborative efforts with schools by contracting with schools to develop identification programs, offering in-service education or developing joint projects pooling the financial resources of the school and the mental health agency.

B. THE REFERRAL PROCESS

A large proportion of child referrals to private practitioners and mental health agencies are usually mediated through the school psychologist, school social worker, or the guidance counselor. These professionals are usually trained in referral procedures. A significant number of referrals are also made directly by teachers and administrators who are not necessarily so trained. With the exception of those exposed to psychotherapy on a personal level or those involved in a counseling training program, they tend to be unaware of the impact of their personal perceptions, attitudes, and beliefs on the referral process.

1. Barriers in Referral Making

Misconceptions concerning therapy that exist in the general population are also present among educators. Such misperceptions and myths range from exaggerated expectations to limited confidence. Among the most common are beliefs that

- Therapy is needed only by the most disturbed;
- Therapy is too long a process to result in immediate changes in school behavior;
- Most emotional problems encountered by students are of a passing nature and will be remedied given sufficient time;
- The school's mission is to educate rather than to become involved in the private lives of students and their families;
- Therapy reduces controls and therefore increases disruptive behavior;

- Therapists perform their work in cloistered offices and rarely communicate with either parents or school personnel;
- Therapists communicate in their own jargon and rarely offer practical recommendations appropriate to the school situation;
- Referral for therapy should not be made before all other methods have been exhausted;
- Most parents would tend to perceive referral as extremely threatening and will therefore resist it. In order to maintain a good relationship between parents and teachers, referrals should be handled by other school professionals; and
- When all other efforts fail, therapy offers the one and only hope for change.

These beliefs are not totally misconstrued. Some are based on reality, while others are due to lack of information about and understanding of the process.

2. Overcoming Barriers to Referral

Both therapists and educators need to change their perspectives and practices in order to address barriers to referral and overcome their impact.

a. The Therapist's Role

Some therapists work in isolation and maintain little communication with other people involved in the child's life. This pattern is due partly to theoretical considerations, namely, the ethics of confidentiality and transferences, and partly to a lack of awareness and skill in the art of collaboration. According to psychoanalytic thinking, transference, a major therapeutic tool, is achieved through close, confidential relationships which must not be diluted. A therapist who enters the role of problem-solver, mediator, or communicator on behalf of the client may tamper with the transference process. Scharff and Scharff (1987), who adopt object relations theory in working with children and families, recognize the significance of transference and countertransference but offer an approach to maintaining open communication within an open system of the family. By focusing on patterns of interaction between family members, the perception of and response of each family member to the therapist and the projections of the whole family toward the therapist, as well as the therapist's feelings and fantasies toward the family and its members, they have defined transference and countertransference as a powerful tool in family therapy.

Therapists of every theoretical orientation need not be deterred from collaborative communication with the family and the school by false notions concerning confidentiality or transference. These need not be tampered with if ethical standards and solid clinical judgment are maintained.

Problems in therapists' communication with schools and families are often inherent in their communication. Some therapists rely on psychological idiom which is often unintelligible or even ominous to those who do not share the language. Others tend to focus solely on the psychodynamics of a problem, ignoring the social context of the child and the family and consequently offering few recommendations relevant to the context.

In order to encourage referrals, therapists can attempt to contact significant personnel at school, work with the family, use language comprehensible to lay personnel, and translate their understanding of the child into practical and relevant recommendations. Maintaining therapist-family-school communication increases the therapist's awareness of the child-family problem. It may result in modification in orientation, strategies and skill and overall effectiveness of the therapy process.

b. The Educator's Role

Educators need help in changing their perspective and beliefs about therapy. Clarification of the following issues may greatly improve understanding and referral practices:

What is therapy? Educators need to be aware of the various models of treating children, such as play therapy, family therapy, behavioral management, cognitive approaches, and group therapy.

How does therapy work? It needs to be pointed out that not all models of therapy are long term. Some are time limited or structured as short-term remediation. Others focus on problem-solving, while others address intrapsychic issues. All models have basic underlying principles and goals. Some principles are shared by all (e.g., the client-therapist relationship, confidentiality, empathy), while others are based on specific theories (e.g., systems theory, learning theory, the role of fantasy and the unconscious, cognitive principles). General understanding of the various stages of therapy may be also helpful.

Who should be referred? Children at risk need to be referred before their problems become extreme. Therapy should not be reserved for the most severe cases and applied only as a last resort. The greater the degree of health, the better chance for healing. Educators need to be aware, however, that not all problems need to be referred for therapy. Differentiation between emotional dysfunction and developmental or cultural issues is essential. Symptom recognition is an important aspect of such differentiation.

What are the communication skills needed in making a referral? Both overt and covert forms of communication play a role in the referral process. On the overt level, educators need skills in communicating to parents in a clear, descriptive language, pointing out the child's strengths and problems. Judgmental language, such as "your child is emotionally disturbed" or "exhibits abnormal behavior," needs to be avoided. Skills are needed in formulating questions that elicit information and cooperation as well as addressing problems openly without raising undue guilt and anxiety.

Awareness of the power of covert communication in making a referral is also important. Fear, reluctance, personal experience all add up to an emotional "package" concerning attitudes toward therapy. These are often communicated to parents as are the more open, direct verbal statements.

How does the therapist have an impact on these attitudes, conceptions, understandings, or misunderstandings? Therapists may consider in-service courses designed to address these issues. Such courses may be offered to a particular school faculty or through a central in-service program for a fee or as a voluntary service, solo or in collaboration with school-based mental health practitioners.

C. ESTABLISHING COLLABORATION

1. Establishing Global Collaboration

Making contact with school personnel to establish collaboration need not be limited to contacts concerning individual cases. It requires a statement of interest on the part of the therapist that she is ready to be involved not only in the issues concerning her clients, but also in the needs of the school as a whole. The following are some of the steps therapists and community agency workers may wish to take to establish a working relationship:

- Identify the school or schools closest to your base of operation;
- Find out the names of the principal, other administrators, guidance personnel, and other mental health school-based professionals;
- Find out about the school-student study team, its leadership, and role;
- Meet with appropriate school personnel to learn about current procedures and practices and express interest in establishing lines of collaboration;
- Offer your services in a variety of areas, including in-service education, consultation, and liaison between school and family.

2. Establishing Case Collaboration

Referrals may be initiated by the school, other agencies (e.g., the courts, child protective services) or may be self-initiated by the family. Most school referrals could usefully be followed by contact with the school.

a. Family-Based Referral

When families initiate referral to a private therapist or an agency, school contact by the therapist may not always be sought by the family. Avoiding the risk of having their child labeled as "problematic," some families seek help without involving the school. In fact, some wish to keep this information completely private. Because parental consent to communication with schools is both legally necessary and therapeutically desirable, therapists need to work with families on issues of withholding information and contact between the therapist and school.

Reluctance to entrust confidential information to school personnel may be associated with a number of issues:

- Fear that the school will be prejudiced against the child because of alleged "emotional problems";
- The fear that information about the student's personal life will be permanently entered into the records;
- The perception of the school as an authoritarian organization which elicits fear and distance. This perception may be associated with personal experiences parents may have had as students;
- The perception of school as an inefficient, poorly structured organization incapable of maintaining appropriate professional and ethical standards;
- The perception of a general adversarial relationship between the family and any bureaucratic organization.

In order to work with families on these issues, a therapist must attempt to differentiate between possible distortions and realistic conditions which justify such attitudes. A local school may, indeed, convey a lack of respect or empathy toward parents or operate nonprofessionally or be lax on matters of confidentiality. However, perceptions that are a function of overgeneralized single experiences, or are due to a general "cautious" orientation toward organizations outside the family or insufficient information, need to be worked through in therapy.

When a cautious parent finally opens up lines of communication with the school, it not only opens the door for increased collaboration between therapist and school, but also enables the family to experience growing trust in the helping potential of organizations outside the family.

With the exception of particularly guarded individuals, most parents, once they understand the benefits that can be derived from collaboration, will grant consent for contact. Those parents who insist on separating the school-therapy entities must, however, be respected in their wish to keep the school-therapy entities separate.

b. School-Based Referrals

Referrals initiated by the school invariably carry the assumption of implicit collaboration. In spite of this assumption, an explicit written consent by the parent or guardian is required before contact is made.

At the initial stages of the referral, it is helpful to find out which school-based professional has been most active in the referral process, let that person know that the referral had been followed through, thank that person for the referral, and establish future liaison with that person.

3. Who Should Be Contacted?

In order to make contact with a school, it is essential to understand the nature of existing lines of communications within a school building. Some schools encourage direct contact between outside practitioners and any member of the school staff. Others tend to designate an individual or group of professionals as liaison to those outside the system. A brief inquiry by phone may help clarify this point. Contact with the school administrator (principal or assistant principal) who is also a "gatekeeper" directing communication and contact may be most useful at this point. The right channel for communication may, therefore, be significantly enhanced not only by following the accepted channels of communication, but also by getting the administrator's backing for the contact. A message from an administrator about the desirability of contact with private practitioners may indeed ease the way to a more direct contact with the appropriate person or persons in the school. It may also open the way to implementation of changes recommended by the therapist.

At the elementary school level, it is usually the classroom teacher who knows the child and the family best. At the secondary level, with increasing program fragmentation, there are usually many professionals involved with the student. Each may hold partial information and possibly have limited interest in the affective aspects of the student's life. It is usually the guidance counselor who holds the key to a more comprehensive knowledge of the student and the family and serves a pivotal role in communication.

Sources of referral and points of contact often originate in school building teams. These teams carry a variety of designations, some of which are Pupil Evaluation Team, Student Study Team, and Pupil Services Team or Pupil Support Team. They usually consist of school mental health staff, health professionals, guidance counselors, special teachers, and administrators. The composition of the teams resembles that of the Committee on Special Education but does not carry its formal and legal characteristics. The teams deal with referrals from teachers, administrators, and counselors and address a variety of student problems. They may make recommendation for further evaluation by a school psychologist, a referral to the Committee on Special Education, as well as specific recommendations to school personnel concerning intervention.

Whether the referral originates with the team or elsewhere, it is important to initiate contact and communicate interest in working collaboratively on the case.

4. A Word of Caution

Feelings of territoriality that exist in most social organizations are also evident in a school structure. They vary in severity, depending on clarity of role definition, degree of confidence experienced by the various groups, and the general level of well-being in the organization. As anxiety increases (e.g., due to budget cuts, major changes in population, or pressures from the community), so do feelings of protectiveness and territoriality. During periods of budgetary pressure, educators, not unlike other workers in other institutions, become extremely wary of others taking on part of their function. Outsiders' collaboration may be perceived as the handwriting on the wall advertising their demise. For example, they may fear that some of the services may be contracted out at the cost of their jobs.

Even during periods of calm and confidence, professionals tend to work within the boundaries defined by the institution, resenting and rejecting invasion by those who "don't belong." This phenomenon tends to intensify during hard times.

Because the introduction of a foreign body (out-of-school professional) into the affairs of a school may be experienced as a threat and violation of boundaries, it is essential for the outside practitioner to be sensitive to this issue, have knowledge of the services offered by a school, and convey respect for their integrity. The outside practitioner does not communicate a purpose and mission to change the school and its practices or attempt to offer services that already exist. Instead, a message of helpfulness, collaboration, and service to both the school and the child must be conveyed.

CHAPTER 6

======

COLLABORATION IN THE ASSESSMENT PROCESS

The assessment process can be significantly enriched through a collaborative effort between the therapist and the school. The data obtained through the process can be potentially useful to the therapist as well as to the teacher and to other school-based personnel. A visit by the therapist to the school can yield important information that is not easily discernible by means of psychological tests or clinical interviews. To obtain a comprehensive picture of the child's patterns of functioning, a school visit should include a field observation, review of school records, and contact with key school personnel.

1. OBSERVING CHILDREN IN A SCHOOL AND IN THE HOME

Observing children in their school environment offers a unique perspective not otherwise available either through an individual contact with the child or by way of contact with the whole family. Observations obtained in an individual interview, in a family setting and in a school situation may be consistent with one another or may offer contradictions. Whether they are mutually reinforcing or contradictory, observing the child in the three context areas, namely, individual, family, and school may yield a more comprehensive and intelligible picture than the one offered by focusing on either one or two of those spheres.

Data concerning the student's behavior can be obtained by means of behavior rating scales completed by teachers. Parents, too, can supply the therapist with behavioral data through informal descriptions, checklists, or rating scales. Information of this nature can be useful to the therapist as it reveals behavior patterns often missed in a one-to-one relationship setting. Such data, however, fail to offer insight into the relationship between observed behaviors in the school setting and its corollaries in the family.

However, with collaboration between therapists, parents, and schools a broader picture of the child's functioning can be gained and some light may be shed on questions such as these:

- Do family interactional patterns repeat themselves in the child's modes of interaction with peers and adults in school?
- Do family communication patterns impact on the child's communication patterns in school?
- Do cognitive modes of behavior in the family have anything to do with the child's learning style at school?

Understanding the *relationship* between home and school functioning can aid immensely in developing appropriate interventions in both situations. Some of the functions that should be observed and compared include the following:

a. Cognitive Functions

Listening

Deficits in listening functions are paramount among children who manifest learning problems. They are usually referred to as Attention Deficit Disorder (ADD).

Attention deficit disorders may be due to problems inherent in the individual's neurological organization or to specific environmental factors, such as poor modeling or an inappropriate sequencing of antecedents and their consequences. It is suggested here that a family systems vantage point may offer an additional perspective on the problem.

Dysfunctional listening behavior in a family system may be a function of numerous dynamic interactions. These may include distance, excessive invasiveness, power struggle, competitiveness, overly rigid boundaries, overly permeable boundaries, or poor communication skills. It can also serve as a message, a metaphor, or a symptom which helps to establish a homeostatic balance.

Viewed from a family systems framework, it may be hypothesized that improved listening behavior in children at school could be achieved through modification of listening behavior in the family.

Organization

Children with learning problems often have difficulty in organization. This is evident in failure to develop appropriate ideational sequencing as well as spatial and temporal concepts.

This difficulty may reflect a deficit within the child, or a familial pattern of organization. Families have their characteristic manner of organizing space, time, possessions, hierarchies, rules, and roles.

Understanding the relationship between the child's mode of organization at school and the family pattern along this dimension may open up new possibilities for intervention. Helping the family improve its ability to organize itself effectively may affect the child's organization at school. Interventions that include family, student, school, and therapist may also have a significant impact on the specific strategies used by children in coping with the learning process.

Conceptualization and Concreteness

Boszormenyi-Nagy and Spark, in their book *Invisible Loyalties* (1973/1984), propose that the ability to learn requires the courage to make a leap from the known to the unknown, from the concrete to the abstract, and that this type of risk taking is only possible through confidence rooted in family relationships.

The ability to move from the concrete to the abstract, from precept to concept, from the specific to the categorical, are the essence of higher learning processes. They are involved in making predictions, classifying and storing information, applying knowledge, making and testing hypotheses, forming judgments and evaluations, and in communicating and sharing ideas.

Individual variability in these functions is not fully understood at this time. The last word is not out yet as to why individuals differ along these lines, or why certain students are more capable of utilizing certain cognitive processes than others.

If we follow Boszormenyi-Nagy's line of thinking, we may turn to the study of family emotional process as a factor in gaining greater understanding of effective learning processes. Questions such as these may be worth exploring:

- What is the relationship between the family's position on the issue of knowing and the child's openness to learning?
- Do secrets in the family interfere with the family and therefore the child's capacity to engage in cognitive exploration?
- Do patterns of emotional impulsivity and a lack of emotional differentiation in the family affect the child's ability to adopt withholding behavior necessary for learning?

Attitudes Toward Learning

To understand children's attitudes toward learning, it may be useful to explore the parallels between the child's observed set of motivations and attitudes and those of the family. Whereas not all attitudes toward learning are inherent in the family situation (as, for example, avoidance of learning tasks that may be associated with failure in this area), the impact of family attitudes is very powerful. Levels of aspiration toward achievement; passivity or involvement in the learning process; openness and a desire to know, alienation, apathy, and resistance all have strong roots in family history. They are transmitted not only through the powerful impact of modeling, but also may reflect multigenerational beliefs. Oppositional behavior on the part of the child expressed as underachievement or misbehavior is often a form of resistance to family or parental values and attitudes.

b. Social and Emotional Functioning

Social and emotional factors affecting children and their families are as significant as cognitive factors in determining children's success or failure at school. In these areas, too, it is useful to view the student's behavior from the vantage point of the school, the family, and the interaction between them.

The following are a number of examples:

Level of Adaptability

Adaptability is considered a major criterion in assessing families. Minuchin (1974) approaches a family assessment by using the rigidity-flexibility continuum and works with families toward increasing their level of adaptability.

It is suggested here that a relationship may exist between the family's level of adaptability and the child's adaptive behavior in learning and in interacting with others.

In assessing student adaptability in a school context, some of the following questions may be considered:

- Can the student shift easily from one activity to another?
- Can the student give and take with others, demonstrating both accommodation and appropriate assertiveness?

- Does the student demonstrate problem-solving ability in the social and cognitive areas?

Observations along this dimension can then be compared with the therapist's assessment of the family along the rigidity-adaptability continuum. In doing so, Minuchin's rigidity-flexibility continuum may be utilized.

Questions such as the following can be raised:

- To what extent are boundaries in the family permeable, rigid, or poorly set?
- To what extent is the family able to shift its problem-solving approach without repeating dysfunctional patterns?
- How powerful are the homeostatic forces that prevent change?
- And, most importantly, to what extent will the child's behavior at school change along with changes in the family along this dimension?

Autonomy and Self-regulation

A student's level of self-regulation and appropriate level of autonomy can also be observed in a school context and in a family setting.

Assessment of a student along this dimension may be guided by the following questions:

- Is the student capable of maintaining momentum at work?
- Can the student work independently for a reasonable duration without excessive reliance on the teacher?
- Does the student generate new solutions to problems?
- Is the student fearful of, accepting of, or overly dependent on authority?

These behaviors can be viewed in light of the student's family interaction along the autonomy and self-regulations issue. The following questions can be explored:

- How is the family characterized with regard to the centrifugal-centripetal continuum?
- To what extent is autonomy encouraged and rewarded?
- Are the family members excessively dependent on each other?
- Is dependency rewarded in the children?

Children may demonstrate similar characteristics at school and at home or may exhibit different behaviors in each context. Consideration of parallels or contradictions and different reactions to different contextual patterns may throw additional light on understanding the child and the family.

c. Level of Anxiety

Bowen (1978), in discussing the role of anxiety in family interaction, believes that assessing levels of family anxiety is essential to determining the level of its functioning. He believes that high levels of anxiety reduce levels of self-differentiation, autonomy, and problem-solving ability. Minuchin also believes that anxiety tends to elevate dysfunctional patterns in the family, and he increases levels of anxiety during family sessions in order to bring dormant patterns to the surface. It is suggested here that the anxiety factor be viewed in a broader context that includes both the school and home environment.

In terms of the school situation, the focus may be placed on the following factors:

- Is anxiety evident in the child through restlessness, lack of self-confidence, shyness, withdrawal, fear of new situations?
- Can the student sustain effort in spite of anxiety?
- How does the student approach the unfamiliar?
- Is the student overly concerned over the quality of his or her work?

Similar patterns of anxiety reactions can be observed in the family:

- Does anxiety in one member of the family reverberate through the system?
- Do family members tend to be overly protective of each other?
- Does the family worry excessively about its image?
- Does the family tend to avoid confronting unfamiliar situations?
- How is anxiety communicated to the children?

Although similar anxiety reactions can be observed both in the child's behavior at school and in the family, it is not unusual to observe a discrepancy in levels of anxiety of the student at home and at school. With a calm school climate, children from anxious families may not manifest excessive anxiety in school. Such a discrepancy may be extremely significant in assessing the relationship between context and symptom. The elements that contribute to calmness at school may be defined and utilized in helping families change.

d. Control and Authority

Issues of power, control, and authority exist in all systems. Parallels may exist along this dimension between the patterns of the student's interaction with peers and teachers and in the student's interaction with parents as well as siblings at home. Although it is useful to observe the child in each setting, it is particularly important to think about the behavior in both systems as a larger system. This perspective may offer data with regard to family control and authority issues as they play themselves out in a school situation. Inconsistencies in relation to this issue also offer significant data.

A number of guiding questions can be kept in mind:

- Does the student appear to be caught up in gaining control over peers and adults?
- Conversely, does the child fail to hold his or her own in social situations?
- Does the child demonstrate leadership ability or is the child essentially a follower?

- To what extent does the child challenge authority, rules, and expectations?
- Is the challenge of authority open or covert?

Similar guiding questions can be asked when the child is seen in a family setting:

- What is the degree of parental control of the children? Do they direct, protect, invade, ignore?
- How do children react to parental power?
- Are the parents involved in a struggle for control with each other?
- What is the degree of consistency or inconsistency in parental exercise of control?

It is particularly significant to observe the extent to which behavioral patterns in the family play themselves out along this dimension at school.

e. Peer and Sibling Interaction

The school situation offers the best opportunity to explore peer interaction and help us to understand them in terms of their family corollaries.

Among the social behaviors worth observing are:

- Level of acceptance of child by others;
- Social roles assumed by children (e.g., child's role as victim, as parent surrogate dispensing moral judgment of peers);
- Combativeness versus cooperation or withdrawal;
- Dependence on approval versus independence; and
- Leadership potential.

In terms of family corollaries, the therapist may observe that sibling relations tend to repeat themselves in the peer relationship context; parent-child interaction patterns may be repeated in the child's attitudes toward the teacher; a child's level of comfort or discomfort in a social group may indeed reflect the family's own sense of comfort or discomfort with its own peer group.

Integrating school and family data enables the therapist to enlarge the therapeutic circle by offering a broader perspective on problems and effecting intervention both at school and in the family.

2. COLLABORATIVE UTILIZATION OF DATA

Collaborative assessment not only involves incorporation of data by utilizing both in-school and out-of-school settings, it also implies therapist-educator collaboration in the assessment process and in the sharing of outcomes.

The observation criteria listed earlier are by no means exhaustive. They are outlined essentially as examples of school behaviors that have corollaries in the family system. Teachers may be able to furnish another set of criteria and thus enrich the therapist observation field.

Teachers, on the other hand, may sharpen their observation and assessment skills by utilizing and incorporating some of the therapist's criteria.

Collaboration in the use of school-family observation data actively involves the family and the child in the assessment process. A family may be guided by the therapist to observe itself and focus on those interactions that contribute toward the child's problems in a school situation. Similarly, the child may be encouraged to focus on his or her role in the problem. In doing so, assessment and intervention overlap as they do in all dynamic systems-oriented approaches to evaluation.

By the process of jointly focusing on the same problem, therapist, educators, parents, and children begin the therapeutic intervention.

3. REVIEWING SCHOOL RECORDS

The school record constitutes the entire body of recorded data on a given student. Portions of the record are usually located at various sites in the school building: guidance office, health office, psychological and social work services, the Committee on Special Education, and local or central district administrative offices. The record includes, among other things, grade transcripts, achievement and cognitive standardized test results, teacher evaluations, parent-teacher conference reports, attendance record, health record, college recommendations, and disciplinary notes. With the exception of grade transcripts, college recommendations and attendance information, the material in the record is confidential. It is available for review or transfer only with written consent by the parent or the former student after the student reaches age 18. Relevant school personnel have direct access to the record. Various safeguards exist in different schools with regard to accessibility of different parts of the record to teachers.

Out-of-school professionals may gain access to the record by obtaining written parental consent or by requesting the parent to obtain copies of parts of the record deemed significant.

Since the record represents a picture of diverse aspects of the child's performance and may be difficult to gather, it is suggested that the therapist focus primarily on relevant portions of the record which are usually kept in the guidance office, the principal's office, or in the school's main office.

The school record offers an historical perspective of the student's growth and development. It may reveal a consistent pattern of performance over the years, or it may present a jagged picture of highs and lows. Comparing such variations with nodal events in the family may shed light on the relationship between such events and school performance.

In addition to the historical perspective, school records need to be examined for other types of information:

1. Measurement and estimates of cognitive potential;
2. Academic standing;
3. Areas of strength and weaknesses;
4. Congruity or incongruity between potential and achievement;

5. Presence or absence of handicapping conditions;
6. Social development; and
7. Health and attendance.

The therapist incorporates information in these areas into the overall assessment picture and adds another dimension to it. The record offers a view of the child as seen and measured by many others. It may serve as a check or a confirmation of the impression gained by the therapist in his or her direct contacts with the child.

The information included in a school record can be a useful tool in helping families address children's problems. Particularly helpful to a family can be increased awareness of the child's characteristics as a learner. The therapist can use the data to help parents set realistic expectations and recognize the child's unique strengths and creative potential. Communicating with school-based personnel may help broaden their perspective of the child in his or her out-of-school context.

4. ASSESSMENT FEEDBACK AND RECOMMENDATIONS

An assessment process is rarely defined as a distinct process, separate from intervention. Systems thinking views assessment and intervention as interwoven and ongoing. When a therapist makes contact with a school to obtain information, the therapist is in fact engaging in an early intervention step. The notion of collaboration is an intervention in and of itself.

Conversely, a conventional diagnostic procedure in a school consists of rather discrete and sequential steps. These include informal information gathering concerning reasons for referrals, basic factual data, observations, formal and informal testing, interpretation of data, and finally reporting. The school mental health professional is involved in carrying out the process, while the teacher and the family are recipients of the product, namely, the results.

Equally important, the therapist, child, and family may help the school personnel become more aware of how school impacts on them wittingly or unwittingly, and perhaps even reinforces the at-risk behavior of the child.

Collaborative assessment is a process characterized by the participation of all parties in the task of learning more about children, their educational needs, and their families. It is a learning process for all involved. The therapist gains a broader perspective, while the teacher learns to sharpen awareness and incorporate ecological-systemic concepts into his or her thinking. It provides for the collaboration in the process of assessment as well as in the product.

CASE EXAMPLE

The following case example will describe ways of using assessment results collaboratively with school personnel.

Joe, a 9-year-old boy, is referred to a private therapist by the school psychologist. The reason for referral is poor academic achievement in spite of high estimated intelligence.

Contact with the school psychologist, school social worker, and review of the record indicate that Joe has had academic problems since first grade. All teachers describe him as poorly focused and inattentive. Reluctance to engage in independent work at school or at home has been a problem for several years. In spite of poor achievement in the major academic areas, Joe has been promoted from grade to grade. Supportive help provided by tutors enabled him to make marginal gains and to avoid a total collapse.

A result of a psychoeducational school evaluation reveals high-average intelligence, a slight fine motor coordination problem, but no major evidence of a learning disability. The school psychologist reports that Joe is "somewhat depressed, has a poor self-image and harbors angry feelings toward his parents."

The school social worker reports that Joe's family is intact. A younger brother is doing well at school. Father is absent from home quite frequently due to his work as a sales representative. Mother is a homemaker and is deeply concerned with her children's welfare. She devotes most of her time to her family and spends many hours helping Joe do his homework. Her parents and other relatives live far away, but there is frequent telephone contact with them. There is little or no contact with members of the father's family.

School medical record reveals an uneventful history.

Joe's teacher describes him as a bright child as evident from his reactions and comments during class discussion. Written output is very limited. The little homework done is achieved by continuous prodding on the part of the teacher and the mother. The teacher and the mother maintain frequent communication to ensure at least a minimal flow of homework. All these efforts result in little improvement. The teacher describes Joe as a "sweet child" who rarely runs into conflict with other children. He is generally agreeable, but it is extremely difficult to get him to do school work.

During the therapist's observation in the classroom, Joe's reluctance to engage in school work was clearly evident. He appeared attentive when an interesting discussion took place but was unable to concentrate on his desk work. At such times he is distracted by arranging papers and pencils, looking for lost objects, or talking to his neighbors. On one occasion, when Joe finally got down to work, he picked up a spelling list which was to be worked on from the top of the list down. Joe began at the bottom of the list and moved up. The order of activities as outlined on the board was also reversed. Instead of following the sequence of math, spelling, and art, Joe followed the sequence of spelling, art, and math (which he failed to complete). It appeared that Joe was setting his own rules concerning the order and conditions. The therapist also noticed that Joe rarely moved from one academic activity to another without the teacher's help. When she was not available to get him started, he withdrew into his desk "puttering." Even though Joe often appeared inattentive, there was evidence that he was listening. His comments suggested that he had been following a point, had retained information, and was using it appropriately. This was true primarily with regard to information presented orally. Reading did not seem to provide a good source of information, as it was too laborious and inefficient. The therapist's impression was that Joe knew what was expected of him but that he was locked into a position that prevented him from functioning.

A family session held around the same time indicated great parental concern over the problem. Both parents appeared to value education a great deal and expressed the desire to offer their children every educational opportunity. Both parents came from a low income background. They both grew up in the same neighborhood and knew each other as teenagers. They were married young when Mrs. S. was 20 and Mr. S. 21. Although they started part-time college attendance, both had to give it up when Mrs. S. became pregnant with Joe. Mrs. S. never returned to her secretarial work, which she held during the first year of her marriage.

Mr. S. earns sufficiently to maintain a small home in a modest neighborhood and provide for the essential needs of the family. However, his income, which is based on commissions, varies from month to month. The family experiences these gyrations as stressful. Mrs. S. and her mother talk on the phone frequently and share information about the children, their health, report cards, and school events. This is in fact the total content of Mrs. S.'s weekly conversations with her mother. Mrs. S.'s mother, who lives on a pension, helps finance some of the tutoring.

Mrs. S.'s youngest brother is developmentally disabled. He lives with his mother in Florida. Mr. S. has little contact with his family of origin. He left home at an early age and made it on his own. During his high school years, he held a variety of part-time jobs and tried not to have to ask his mother for support. Believing that she had more than her share of trouble dealing with his alcoholic father, he did not wish to add to the burden. When she died, his contact with his family ceased.

In family session, Joe and his brother sat close to their mother and watched her signals before talking. Both children remained rather quiet during the session, while Mrs. S.

did most of the talking. Although Joe appeared inattentive, it was obvious that he was listening to every word.

The parents, and particularly Mrs. S., described the family as close and happy except for the turmoil caused by Joe's school work. Homework time turns into a daily battleground. Mother cajoles, helps, awards, and punishes, while Joe turns off. These sessions often end up in angry explosions between Joe and his father. Mother interferes, tries to stop the fighting, and determines to take over the job with greater patience. In spite of all the efforts, Joe continues to hold back on doing his work.

The therapist begins to form a number of hypotheses concerning the function of Joe's symptoms.

The learning problem exhibited at school and at home is not characteristic of either cognitive deficit, a learning disability, physical problems, or an attention deficit. Although cognitive style is essentially auditory, there is no evidence that the problem is rooted in perceptual or processing deficits. The teacher demonstrates a high degree of sensitivity and support to Joe and his family. The therapist forms the impression that Joe's approach to learning tasks is essentially negativistic. He rejects assignments made by others but chooses his own conditions and rules under which he will learn. Even though Joe does not appear to be rebellious (in fact he appears very compliant during family sessions and at school), he is most noncompliant when it concerns school work. The therapist reaches a tentative hypothesis that Joe's problem is rooted in a power struggle between him and the significant authority figures in his life.

The exploration of the dynamics behind this struggle is open for further study and intervention in the future.

At this junction, it is important to offer feedback to the family and child and to the school. Interpretation of data may be discussed with small subsystems such as the family or school personnel. It may also take the form of a conference that includes family-student-educators and therapist.

The results of a student and family assessment are never final. The assessment picture changes with changing environmental conditions, developmental factors, and the assessment process in and of itself. It often represents the first breakthrough in a stagnant situation and often an opportunity for change. The hope experienced by children, families, and school personnel during the assessment process is often an opportune time to bring greater flexibility into the school-child-family interaction.

Conversely, if assessment is not accompanied or followed by meaningful intervention, it often represents another dead end in the history of all involved. Unfortunately, the latter situation occurs much too often due to time pressures, shortage of support personnel, and fragmentation of services. Collaborative efforts within the school and between the school-family-child-therapist can greatly facilitate a productive utilization of the assessment data. The next steps in the collaborative effort following the assessment will be discussed in the next chapter.

CHAPTER 7

COLLABORATION IN FEEDBACK, TREATMENT PLANS, AND FOLLOW-UP

1. COLLABORATION IN ASSESSMENT FEEDBACK

Feedback to the school at the "completion" of the assessment process may lay the groundwork for further collaboration. It should be addressed to all school personnel who were involved in the information gathering process, namely, the classroom teacher, mental health professionals, appropriate specialists (e.g., reading, speech), and interested administrators. The reporting process may be carried out along the following lines:

a. Description of process as assisted by various school personnel;
b. Summary of school-based data;
c. Summary of out-of-school data;
d. Additional feedback by school personnel;
e. Tentative interpretation of problem as based on school and out-of-school data; and

121

f. Tentative collaborative goal setting for the direction of treatment as seen by the therapist and by school personnel.

An evaluation feedback conference that includes the total system—school, family, student, and therapist—is perhaps the most conducive to collaboration and successful treatment. Such a conference conveys the message that there are no guilty parties who carry the burden of the child's problems. Instead, there is a coalescing of the most significant persons in the child's life, all attempting to find solutions acceptable and helpful to all.

Furthermore, such a meeting conveys a message of caring, of doing things out of the ordinary routine to make things work.

There are a number of other advantages to this format:

a. In the presence of the child, the family, all professionals, be they school-based or out-of-school, must adopt a pragmatic language that will be intelligible to all. Such communication tends to reduce fatal language expressions that carry heavy judgmental tones.

b. All participants have a chance to respond and add to the interpretation as they see fit. The child and the family, therefore, are active participants rather than passive recipients. All participants may feel empowered by the therapist when their feedback is sought, respected, and incorporated into the total picture.

c. All participants hear the same message. Although individuals may not all interpret the content of the discussion in the same way, this format reduces the level of distortion. It is therefore important to summarize each person's understanding of the message.

d. It encourages commitment on the part of the parent, child, school personnel, and therapist to enter into a therapeutic contract.

2. FORMULATING TREATMENT PLANS

The content of the feedback conference may vary with the therapist's orientation and his or her specific dynamic interpretation. The basic message, however, needs to help the child, family, and school give and receive information which will enable them to modify their behavior.

For a collaborative treatment plan to be effective, it must be congruent with school practices and realistically incorporated into the school program. A therapist may formulate a plan compatible with the assessment of the problem and yet find it incompatible with existing conditions in the school. Without proper conditions for implementation, a plan may be clinically sound but may be impractical if the school either rejects the plan or proceeds in a contradictory direction. However, if school personnel participate in formulating the plan, they may accept suggestions more easily or may even suggest modifications in school procedure that may help the child. Such modification may be generalized to benefit other children.

The following are two examples dealing with collaborative formulation of treatment plans, each based on the case of Joe described on pages 115 to 119.

One example demonstrates the advantages and pitfalls in formulating a system-based approach, and the other demonstrates the same from a behavioral perspective.

CASE EXAMPLE: SYSTEMS-ORIENTED APPROACH

In the case of Joe, the therapist views Joe's "underachievement" as a function of a family interaction. She observes that not only is Joe locked in a battle for control with his mother, but that control and power issues underlie all relationships in the nuclear family. Conflict over the "rightness" of one's position exists between the parents, parents and children, siblings, and even extend to relationships with grandparents and other members of the extended family. The therapist further observes that the control issue is expressed not only through frequent criticism and confrontations but also through benevolent behavior. This is evident in the mother's deep commitment to her role, her anxiety about her children's welfare, and her continuous vigilance.

Adding systemic thinking to her repertoire, the clinician may decide to explore the marital relationship and its relationship to the excessive involvement of the mother. She may choose to approach the problem as an intergenerational pattern of parent-child interaction, focusing on the dysfunctional hierarchical problem. She may address the issue utilizing a cognitive dimension that examines the beliefs and myths which support the control issue. Regardless of the particular direction adopted by the therapist, most systems-oriented therapists would seek to reduce control and overinvolvement and help the family to develop more appropriate hierarchical delineations that permit a balance between autonomy and nurturance.

The therapist is poignantly aware of the challenge confronting the family. She knows that it would be extremely difficult for an overly responsible parent to take a backstage position or permit the other parent to actively enter the picture. She also knows that a great deal of anxiety will be experienced in the process of change. The mother's anxiety may increase as she is watching her child be exposed to possible temporary failure and pain.

The difficulty for the family may be reduced and the achievement of therapeutic goals accelerated when support from other sources (e.g., extended family, friends, school) is available.

On the other hand, progress may be impeded in the presence of forces that negate the process. Thus, a school's insistence that the mother take charge and ensure full compliance with homework assignments may be in total conflict with the therapeutic goal for the mother to be less involved at this time and may endanger the therapeutic process.

A collaborative understanding and formulation of treatment goals and plans may avert unnecessary hurdles. Parents, school, therapist, and student need to be working together toward the same goal, namely, that of empowering Joe to make choices, confront his own errors, acquire appropriate autonomy, and learn to assume responsibility. This goal can only be achieved if all parties understand the problem and agree on a common direction.

Not all teachers may be able to cooperate with a "hands off" policy regardless of how short term it may be. The difficulty may be rooted in a different ideology or in the teacher's perception of her role.

Although the school's mission, policies, and practices are indeed different from those set by the therapist, the notion of collaboration may nevertheless be possible. In the case of Joe, for instance, the school may continue to make its own demands on Joe but without pulling the parent into the process. Joe will pass or fail strictly on the basis of what goes on between him and his teacher.

Paradoxically in this case, collaboration may call for a lesser parent-teacher partnership on the issue of work.

CASE EXAMPLE: BEHAVIORALLY ORIENTED THERAPY

A behavior therapist may approach Joe's problem differently. But this therapist, too, will need to gain the cooperation of the school and consider the limitations inherent in such collaboration.

The therapist may observe that the reward/punishment balance in the family weighs heavily in the direction of punishment—that Joe is becoming habituated to punishment and becoming oblivious to parental interventions. The therapist sets as a treatment goal the altering of the relationship between Joe's behavior and its consequences. Instead of reliance on punitive measures, the family will be coached in applying rewarding consequences for desired behavior. This approach requires consistency in applying the strategy at home as well as consistency between school and home. If the parents follow the approach but the teacher employs essentially punitive methods, the course of change may be seriously jeopardized. It is, therefore, essential that both parents and school professionals understand the rationale behind the therapeutic plans and commit themselves to collaboration during its implementation.

3. IMPLEMENTING THE TREATMENT PLAN

The usefulness of the family-school-student-therapist conference was discussed earlier in the context of assessment. It can also be an effective tool in the process of intervention. To best illustrate the utilization of this procedure, reference will be made again to the case of Joe. As mentioned earlier, Joe is a bright 9-year-old who achieves poorly and is minimally motivated to engage in school work. The therapist believes that Joe is locked into a power struggle with his parents and that structural family dynamics are at the core of the problem. She sets as the therapeutic goal the restructuring of the power organization and the intensity of emotional involvement in the family. She attempts to effect a change by helping the mother shift her overresponsible position as a parent and become involved with issues concerning her own person, increase contact and communication between Joe and his father, encourage Joe to make a choice with regard to success or failure at school and encourage the parents to plan more activity together as a couple.

In addition to ongoing family sessions around these issues, the therapist may also set a collaborative conference with the school. This conference may be instrumental in enhancing Joe's ability to take control in a more productive fashion than his current passive resistance.

Specific modes of intervention vary with the orientation of the therapist. However, a consistency of approach between school and home is of great value.

In the case of Joe, the following intervention strategies may be carried out collaboratively by family and the school:

a. Joe's homework is strictly in the realm of the student-teacher territory. The teacher (not the parent) will check the homework and will take appropriate measures to encourage productivity.
b. Joe's father will get involved in helping only if Joe requests such help.
c. Father will inform Joe about his availability and Joe will seek out help only during those times.
d. Mother will be encouraged to take a partial "vacation" from her homework responsibility, since she had already completed her own schooling. She might, however, pursue activities in areas of personal interest to her.
e. The teacher will contact the family when necessary rather than set a regular weekly reporting procedure. Joe will be informed on the content of the teacher's message to the family.

4. FOLLOW-UP

Since most interventions are, in essence, probes based on limited observations and tentative hypotheses, their validity needs to be checked through feedback and follow-up. School personnel may be instrumental in helping the therapist check outcomes. If school personnel and family report successful outcomes as anticipated, the therapist gains greater confidence in the accuracy of the hypothesis and effectiveness of the intervention. If, however, anticipated outcomes fail to occur, modification may be necessary either in reformulating the diagnostic hypothesis, in the implementation of specific interventions, or in designing different change strategies.

Brief telephone contact with the classroom teacher and the mental health professionals at critical points are very helpful indeed in both reinforcing and evaluating change strategies and in maintaining them on the agreed upon ongoing targets. School personnel should also be encouraged to contact the therapist any time they see fit.

5. CONCLUSION: LIMITS TO COLLABORATION

Collaboration does not necessarily mean that family, school, and therapist have identical views on the nature of the problem and the means to achieve change. Although all seek the child's welfare, they differ somewhat in the perception of their mission in promoting the child's optimal growth.

Families are committed, among other values, to the transmission of tradition, beliefs, continuity, cohesiveness, survival, procreation, and nurturance. Educators are committed to the transmission of specific bodies of knowledge, values, and skills, while the therapist is committed, essentially, to helping clients achieve optimal growth and freedom from dysfunctional patterns in behaviors and interactions.

Because of these differences in emphasis, educators, therapists, and parents may differ on many issues. These include permissiveness and control, adult supervision, autonomy, locus of control and initiative, aggression and passivity, attitudes toward authority, competition, affiliation, and many others.

In addition to such differences in focus, families, schools, and therapists operate under different conditions. Although the therapist and the family may work to see more individualization of instruction for the child, the teacher's specific classroom situation may prevent him or her from collaborating on this point. It is not the goal of collaborative therapy to set identical goals for all, nor is the goal for all parties to move in lockstep fashion. Rather, it is the facilitation of respect for each set of unique goals and the cross-fertilization of ideas that constitute the essence of collaboration, leading to workable plans.

Chapters 8 and 9 will present two case studies that demonstrate the collaboration models described in Chapters 5, 6, and 7.

CHAPTER 8

MULTIPLE SIBLING PROBLEM: A CASE OF THERAPIST- FAMILY-SCHOOL COLLABORATION

The collaboration models described in Chapters 3, 4, 5, 6, and 7 may appear complex and labor intensive. However, great savings can occur through the use of a collaborative model if duplication of services are reduced, if communication between various services is enhanced and, above all, if all participants involved in the case sense the power and value of their contribution.

The following case is an example of collaboration involving a family with three children who demonstrated difficulty at school.

BACKGROUND

The Gordon family lives in a middle-class suburb in the Northeast. The father, Stan, is age 45, the mother, Laura, is age 42, Jeff is age 16, Alex is age 14, and Ben is age 12.

A. The Referral

Mrs. Gordon called the private therapist to set up an appointment for her son, Alex. Her call came at the recommendation of the school counselor. Recently Alex had been having repeated conflicts with teachers, which resulted in in-school and out-of-school suspensions. While inquiring about the rest of the family, the therapist learned that both the younger and the older boys were having behavioral and learning problems, but that they were less severe. The mother thought she could handle their problems on her own. The therapist suggested that the whole family come in for the first session, and the suggestion was willingly agreed upon. The therapist also asked Mrs. Gordon for written permission to contact school personnel to review school records if necessary.

The guidance counselor of the middle school where Ben and Alex were enrolled was contacted by the therapist to inform her of the referral and to obtain information concerning the children's school behavior. The guidance counselor reported that of the two brothers, Alex was having the greater difficulty at school. He was running into conflicts with teachers, often talking back to them, walking out of the classroom without permission, and refusing to participate in class work. Homework was poorly executed and often missing. Ben also had problems doing school work. He often "shut down" and refused to do any work. In addition, he occasionally "exploded." The guidance counselor also intimated that she had known Jeff when he was in the middle school and that he, too, had had trouble. The counselor informed the therapist that a building pupil service committee was scheduled to meet in the near future and that more specific information would be available then. She was planning to schedule both students on the agenda. The therapist made arrangements through the school administration to attend that meeting.

B. School Assessment

Due to program compartmentalization in the middle school, it was not possible to observe the boys in the actual classroom setting. However, information from teachers was conveyed through the study team.

1. The Building Study Team Conference

The following school personnel were present: school dean (chair), guidance counselor, school psychologist, school social worker, and the educational evaluator. The teachers participated through the written notes that they sent to the guidance counselor.

Dean's report. Alex is being sent frequently to the dean's office due to misbehavior. He uses foul language with teachers and has left the room abruptly and without permission several times. During the last incident he used expletive language toward a teacher and was suspended from school for three days. During a disciplinary conference held by the dean with Alex and his parents, it was decided that Alex would modify his behavior and that progress notes would be sent by teachers to the dean weekly. An evaluation conference with the dean is scheduled in another month. Ben has not been referred to the dean, but earlier discussions of the building team indicated that the case needs further attention.

School psychologist's report. Alex has had behavior problems since the early grades. In grade 2 he was referred to the Committee on Special Education and was classified as emotionally disturbed. He was placed in a special education program during grades 3 through 5. He did well in the program, was returned to regular middle-school classes, and was declassified by the Committee on Special Education. The report completed by the elementary school psychologist indicates that recommendations were made for psychotherapy. The middle-school psychologist recommended that the case be reopened with the Committee on Special Education and that a current psychological evaluation be undertaken.

Social worker's report. The school social worker had been in touch with Mrs. Gordon over the year. She described Mrs. Gordon as a conscientious, hard-working parent who is often overwhelmed by her children's demands. Her husband is absent much of the time, trying to hold on to the family business, which is on the verge of collapse. She suffers from frequent migraine headaches. Attempts at getting psychotherapy for Alex were made in the past, but they were unsuccessful because Alex refused to see a therapist. Mrs. Gordon felt that she could not add the burden of getting Alex to therapy to all the other responsibilities she carried.

Guidance counselor's report. The counselor had had personal contact with both Alex and Ben. Alex was usually angry at his teachers and openly claimed that he did not want to cooperate. However, following such protestations he calmed down for a few days. Alex is a talented singer and actor and got along well with the drama teacher. He had major roles in school productions. He is also a good athlete and is socially accepted. Ben was quieter and does not create much fanfare, but he, too, had left the classroom in a huff, refusing to listen, participate, or take tests. Unlike his brother, Alex, he did not curse at adults. Ben is a good athlete, but he often refused to change his clothes at gym and had been expelled from athletic activities due to noncompliance. Teachers' reports indicate that most of the teachers believed the boys to be more capable than their performances showed. Both were weak in the language areas. Ben did better in science and mathematics than in English and social studies. Descriptions of the boys' behavior were consistent with the other reports.

Team's recommendations (including the therapist). Permission would be obtained from the parent to perform preliminary psychoeducational evaluations by the psychologist and the educational evaluator. Alex's case needed to be reopened with the Committee on Special Education. Whether Ben should be referred to the Committee on Special Education would be determined at the completion of the preliminary testing. The purpose of the evaluation was to determine the following:

a. To assess to what extent learning deficits, especially in language-related areas, affected the performance of Alex and Ben;
b. To obtain personality profiles and assess the role of emotional issues underlying the problems;
c. To determine whether family issues were interfering with the boys' ability to function at school.

Other recommendations made were:

a. The social worker would meet with Mrs. Gordon and help in management and parenting issues.
b. The counselor would hold frequent sessions with each of the boys and try to enable them to "vent" their feelings away from the classroom.
c. The therapist would assess the family dynamics. At this point in the meeting the therapist explained some of the methods used in the evaluation and the constraint of confidentiality. Information concerning the needs of the boys at school would be open for mutual discussion but personal information concerning the family members would not be communicated.
d. The therapist would be in frequent contact with the school. The guidance counselor would be the contact person. Once the evaluation procedures were complete and the family was committed to a therapeutic course of action, contacts would be less frequent. However, the school or the therapist might initiate contact at any time, as needed.

2. *School Records*

Alex and Ben entered the current school system in kindergarten. Narrative teachers' reports were summarized in the guidance counselor's report. Health and attendance records were normal. However, they point to a "see-saw" pattern of behavioral difficulty. When Ben was having major problems, Alex was more contained; when Alex was having major problems, Ben was more contained.

Academic achievement as portrayed by grades was very uneven for Alex. His grades ranged from B to D to F without a consistent pattern regarding either teacher or subject. The grades changed dramatically within a given year as well as from year to year.

Ben showed a definite preference for mathematics and science, in which he received better grades and better achievement test results than in language arts. Reading and writing skills were acquired slowly but not poorly enough to require special education.

Resistance to homework was indicated repeatedly. Teachers, in their narratives, used more sympathetic language in depicting Ben as compared to Alex. They described Ben as sensitive, friendly, and intelligent but as unmotivated and a poor achiever. Alex is described as angry, sullen, unpredictable, creative, and intelligent.

Arrangements were also made to review Jeff's records. Since Jeff's problems were not urgent at that time, it was decided that the therapist would call the guidance counselor at the high school and ask her cooperation in reviewing the records together over the telephone. A copy of Mrs. Gordon's permission to communicate with the school went out to the counselor, and an appointment was set for a telephone conversation. The counselor was open to such communications because she had had some questions regarding Jeff, who appeared to her to be "a very unhappy child."

Jeff was described by the counselor as a "good looking" and hard-working young man. Teachers had always described him as conscientious, well liked by peers, and active in athletics. His achievement, as compared to the effort he made, was below expectation. Grades were in the C to D range. He had been classified by the Committee on Special Education as learning disabled since grade 5. He was given resource room services, which he still used for purposes of receiving a waiver on time limits on tests. No particular behavior problems were evident at that time. Jeff was myopic but wore corrective glasses. No other health issues were reported.

3. Therapist's Review

In reviewing the material gathered through the records and the school team meeting, the therapist began to make a few initial observations and set forth questions to be considered in the near future. These were as follows:

a. All three children have had varying degrees of difficulty. The language areas, and particularly writing, was a common deficit in all three. Is there a common or similar learning disability affecting all of them?

b. Completion of homework assignments was a problem for all the children. What was the relationship between the writing problems they had and completing written work? Was there a specific deficit that affected motivation or did emotional and motivational problems interfere with productivity?

c. Two of the three boys had relationship problems with authority figures. Peer relations appeared normal.

d. Each of the youngsters, and particularly the two younger ones, took the center stage almost in synchrony, each occupying it at any given time. (In her call Mrs. Gordon referred to this phenomenon as "taking turns." The school was not aware of this pattern since they were dealing with each of the boys as a separate case.) Did this pattern have any significance?

e. What was under the eruption of symptoms at that time after a period of relative calm? Were there changes either in the school or home environment that were throwing things off balance?

f. What were the family issues being communicated and expressed through the boys' attitudes? The therapist kept these observations and questions in mind for further exploration.

C. The Therapist's Evaluation of the Family

1. First Session

At the suggestion of the therapist, the whole nuclear family attended the first session. Present were the father, Stan; the mother, Laura; and sons Jeff, Alex, and Ben. The family arranged itself into a semicircle with Stan and Laura at the extremes and the boys in the middle. Ben was sitting close to Laura, often leaning on her and watching her clues. Jeff sat near his father, and Alex was in the middle.

They understood that the purpose of the meeting was to help Alex get along better at school. The parents both agreed that he was difficult to reach because he exploded before they had a chance to talk to him. His leaving the scene when he was angry posed a real problem in communication. Jeff offered the observation that his younger brothers were "brats" and that the parents did not handle them correctly. He felt that they should be better disciplined and punished. Jeff felt that he was the one good and helpful child in the family. He was the only one who helped Mother in trying to stop the other two from fighting. He expressed the feeling that it did not pay to be good because no one either paid attention or appreciated it. He might as well not try. Laura introjected at that point by saying that she had asked him many times not to do her job as a parent, but he kept doing it.

Alex said little at the session. He looked sullen, with his eyes directed to the floor much of the time. When approached directly, he would shrug and say, "I don't know."

Ben said he hated sharing a room with his brother because of the fighting that went on all the time.

Stan and Laura also felt that Alex was the one with the most problems. When asked about their opinion concerning other people in the family, Laura intimated that all the boys had had academic and behavioral problems at school at one time or another. Stan agreed with Laura.

Parenting roles were pretty well set. Stan saw his responsibilities as a provider, and he worked hard at it. With the children he acted primarily in a disciplinary role. He was not happy having to do that, but he felt that he must do so because his wife was too lax. His parents were strict with him, and he believed that they did a good job rearing him and his sister. Laura felt overwhelmed with her parental responsibilities and wished Stan would spend more fun time with the boys. All three boys shared the same wish. Jeff expressed the desire to have more to do with his father and also for the family to be doing more things together.

The therapist focused on the problems of the family as a whole. It was agreed that there were issues in the family that could be worked out. All participants, except Alex, agreed to return and to work on their interrelationships.

2. Second Session

The second session was scheduled with Stan and Laura alone in order to gain understanding of the couple relationship and to set the stage for the development of greater cohesion in the couple both as parents and as spouses.

A history of the marital couple was obtained. Stan grew up in the town where the family now lives. He attended the same schools. His parents were relatively well to do, as his father owned and quite successfully managed a small clothing manufactory. Stan has a younger sister who is married and lives with her husband and two children in another state. When Stan's parents retired, they offered him the management of the business, which he accepted and is still managing. His business is not doing as well because of competition with imported goods. He often thinks of selling it, but does not know what he can do instead. He also believes that he would have to sell at a considerable loss and actually give away the business his father developed and entrusted to him. Stan attended two years of college and dropped out to take over the business. He did not do well either in college or in high school. He remembers always being jumpy, having trouble concentrating, and being endowed with a very poor memory.

Laura grew up in the same town. She excelled in school and earned a scholarship to go to college. She attended a college out of town for one semester but felt so lonely and homesick that she returned and completed her studies at a local university. She acquired a degree teaching home economics. She taught in a junior high school for two years before the children were born. She is well groomed and has an outgoing manner. Laura comes from a lower middle-class family and considered herself part of "the other side of the tracks."

As a youngster, her clothes were not always consistent with the acceptable style, and her home was poorly furnished. She has a younger brother who was her main companion as a child. He developed drug abuse problems in later life and moved to another state. She has no contact with him now. As a youngster she also had no friends her own age because she was very quiet and believed to be strange because of her unfashionable clothes and her chubbiness. She spent much time with her mother, who rarely left the house because of many phobias and feelings of being out of place in the community. Her father was a gentle person, and she felt close to him. He worked as a postal clerk and did not think much of his ability to earn money. Laura remembers her childhood as lonely and depressing. She feels depressed now just thinking about it.

Stan's family welcomed Laura with open arms. They believed that she would influence their son to be more studious and stable. After they were married, Laura and Stan spent much of their free time visiting Stan's parents. Stan's mother took Laura on shopping trips and pretty much determined what she would wear. She also tried to educate Laura on matters of household management and home decorating. For the first few years Laura enjoyed this type of attention. It was in sharp contrast with her childhood lifestyle.

Laura and Stan gradually curtailed their contacts with Laura's family. When Laura's father died, her mother moved away to the sun belt. Looking back, Laura feels that she was too dazzled by Stan's family's generosity. She regrets not having realized the price she paid in choosing his family over her own—the price being headaches, alienation, and loneliness.

Things began to change for Laura after Jeff was born. She was beginning to resent her mother-in-law's benevolent interference, as she wanted to try her hand as a mother. Conflicts ensued, but Stan's mother's behavior did not change. Laura became more assertive toward her mother-in-law. She felt resentful over her husband's failure to stand up to his parents and his continuous need to maintain close daily contact with them. Until this very day, Stan's first activity when he returns home is a telephone call to his father to discuss the business of the day.

After Alex's birth Laura developed severe headaches which continue to plague her. She places the responsibility for her unhappiness on Stan because he distances from her and the boys. When he does become involved, he usually yells and disciplines them. He often gets into rages with them at which time he yells uncontrollably and then leaves the room. Laura feels intimidated by these explosions and vows not to involve him in the children's discipline. However, sometimes things become too overwhelming for her and she tries to involve him, usually with predictable results.

Stan views his temper as problematic, but he feels that he has his reasons to be angry. Laura, in his opinion, is very inconsistent and lets the children go wild when she has a headache (which is often). The house is also in disarray. He wishes Laura would "get a hold of her life."

It was obvious to the couple and to the therapist that many problems existed in the couple's relationship as well as in the coordination of their roles as parents. It was not difficult to help them see that they needed help as a couple and that the family as a whole, and not only Alex, should be the focus of further therapy.

3. Third Session

This session was held with the whole family. The main focus was the articulation of the goals for treatment and to formulate the therapeutic contract. Each member was asked to identify the changes he or she would like to see in the family relationship. They responded as follows:

- *Jeff* wants less fighting between the boys and between the parents and more activities for the family as a whole. Jeff fears that the parents may divorce. He wants to do all he can to keep the family together. For himself he wants more quiet at home and more time to spend with his father fishing or playing ball.
- *Alex* wants to be left alone. He resents Jeff getting on his case and Ben for following the same behavior. He had difficulty articulating other needs.
- *Ben* also wants time alone with his father. He would like his father to watch his computer games.
- *Laura* wants Stan to "enter the family," come home earlier in the evening, listen to the children, help them with their homework, and show interest in their work. She would like to have the family eat together more often. She wants Stan to be less temperamental with the boys and not criticize her in front of them. She would like to have some time for herself and not to be at the beck and call of the children and the school at all times.
- *Stan* wants the boys to fight less, do their homework on their own, and behave in school. As for Laura, he would like to see her be more in control.

None of the members of the family were able, at that time, to articulate needs for change in terms of their own responsibilities. Each was expecting the others to change. This is not unusual for a family starting in therapy. They had moved, however, from focusing solely on Alex to recognizing family issues to which they were willing to attend.

4. Therapist's Initial Thoughts Concerning the Family Strengths

In spite of perpetual conflict, the family seeks greater cohesiveness. Readiness to seek solutions to better relationships is expressed by all. Furthermore, Laura and Stan recognize that their marital relationship is in trouble, and they are willing to work toward its improvement.

Areas of vulnerability. Stan and Laura seem to have had difficulty establishing their own boundaries as a couple. Moving into the role of "children" with Stan's parents, they did not have an opportunity to let their own relationship work out its highs and lows. Stan's continuing excessive attachment to his family of origin and Laura's separation from her own leaves them with unresolved developmental issues.

Both Stan and Laura have questions concerning their own competencies. Laura questions Stan's competency as a parent while he questions his own ability to make ends meet for the family. Laura feels quite defeated in her parental role, a situation that is reinforced by Stan's criticism. The spouses are not aware of the extent to which they exacerbate each other's sense of incompetence.

The children's symptoms may have several functions, one of which might be to get attention in a family where there is not enough support to go around. Each of the children is taking his turn for attention when the others are less demanding. The children may also be signaling the total family's trouble, challenging the status quo. In this setting, perhaps Alex is either being set up or is setting himself up as the scapegoat.

Parental modeling, especially with regard to the expression of anger, reinforces explosiveness and "walking out of the field" when anger becomes overwhelming. The father and two of the boys walk out in protest when angry and the mother gets migraine headaches and disappears.

An imbalance (or perhaps balance) exists between Stan and Laura with regard to their involvement with the boys. Stan is underinvolved while Laura is overinvolved. Perhaps the behavior of one is a function of the other.

These issues and others that are likely to emerge will constitute the essence of the therapist's intervention with the family.

D. The School Psychological Evaluation

Although the various aspects of the assessment are presented sequentially, some of the assessment activities were carried out simultaneously. The psychoeducational evaluation was conducted at the school, while the therapist was making her initial assessment away from school.

As agreed during the school study team conference, testing was to be administered with both Alex and Ben. Parental approval was obtained easily. The high school counselor indicated to the therapist that psychological testing at the school would not be carried out for Jeff because at that time there were no serious manifestations of problems at school. Most of Jeff's problems were manifested at home.

1. Test Results on Alex

The following tests were administered: Wechsler Intelligence Scale for Children-Revised (WISC-III); Wechsler Individual Achievement Scale (WIAT); and projective techniques. On the WISC-III Alex obtained a high average score on the Verbal Scale (Verbal IQ 115) and average score on the Performance Scale (Performance IQ 104). His Full Scale IQ was 111. The highest subscores were achieved on the Information, Vocabulary, and Comprehension tests, while the lowest scores were in Coding and Picture Arrangement. The overall picture indicated that verbal and mathematical competencies were the most prominent, while motor-visual and space organization skills fell below average. On the WIAT, Alex achieved the highest score in Reading, Mathematical Reasoning, and Numerical Operations. Lowest scores were in Listening Comprehension, Written Expression, and Spelling. The cognitive tests point to good intellectual potential as well as skill to enable Alex to achieve well in most academic areas. However, he is poorly organized, lacks attentional skills, and produces far below expectation levels in all academic areas where writing is required.

Projective tests reveal poor impulse control, considerable anger, poor self-image, and lack of trust in the significant adults around him.

2. Test Results on Ben

Ben was administered the WISC-III, the Woodcock-Johnson Achievement Test-Revised, the Bender Gestalt, the Slingerland Screening Test for Identifying Children with Specific Language Disability, and projective tests.

On the WISC-III Ben achieved an IQ score of 123 (superior range) with a Verbal IQ score of 116 (high-average range), and a Verbal Scale IQ of 122 (superior range). Ben's greatest strength showed up in verbal reasoning, verbal comprehension, abstract reasoning, and vocabulary. Lowest scores emerged on tests that require visual vigilance, speed, accuracy, and motor-visual organization.

On the achievement test the highest scores were obtained in reading, reading comprehension, math calculation, as well as problem solving. Lowest levels were achieved in spelling and in writing. Motor control on all written tests was immature.

The Slingerland test identified difficulty in converting auditory stimuli into writing.

The Bender Gestalt indicated difficulty in organization and poor motor control.

Projective tests revealed a picture of a rather depressed child who views himself as inadequate and fragile. Emotionally he is holding onto patterns of dependency typical of younger children. Anger and anxiety were quite prevalent.

E. Combining School and Family Data

When the therapist considered the total data obtained at school and in the therapist's office, a number of major conclusions occurred.

a. Writing difficulties are evident for all three siblings and the substantiation of a motor-visual and organizational problem in more recent tests appear to constitute a familial disability. Considering the father's school history, there is a possibility that a constitutional factor is involved. Regardless of its origin at this point, direct remediation in this area is indicated.

b. The disability may be partly responsible for the poor self-image and motivational difficulty in doing written work (mostly homework). However, family issues seem to be playing a very powerful role in the dysfunction. These included lack of consistent support and limit setting; inappropriate expression of anger; anxiety related to parental conflict; competition for attention; unfinished business between each parent and his or her parents, with the result being delayed maturation in the parental and marital roles; and the possibility that each sibling is taking on the scapegoat role intermittently.

c. It was evident that the factors in the above points (a and b) act upon each other, thus perpetuating and aggravating the symptoms, leaving the children and the parents stuck in their problems.

F. Feedback and Recommendations: School Conferences

Following the completion of the evaluation process, separate conferences were held in the school for Alex and for Ben. The following individuals attended: the parents, the student, the guidance counselor, the school psychologist, and the private therapist.

The school psychologist reported the results of the tests in simple language. She emphasized to each of the children that the tests proved what the teachers and parents had observed; namely, that they had good learning ability. It was also indicated that they had academic strengths as well as weaknesses. The particular strengths and weaknesses were pointed out to each student. The school psychologist and the guidance counselor both suggested that the problem was not due to an inability to learn but to the attitudes and particular methods with which they approached their work.

The following recommendations were made:

a. The service of a writing teacher would be offered. This service could be obtained through the Committee on Special Education (CSE) or directly through participation in the writing lab program. The advantages of both options were discussed. Both Alex and Ben opted for the writing lab even though it offers less time than did the daily assistance of a resource-room teacher for special education. The parents also opted for this approach. It was decided to offer the writing lab service on an experimental basis. If the service was found to be insufficient, a resource-room teacher would be considered by way of the CSE.

b. If either boy failed to produce assigned homework, the school would deal with the problem internally by means of grading penalties, detention, or loss of free-time activities.

c. The parents agreed to become involved in homework only if requested by the children. The children would be reminded of their schedules, but would not be cajoled, reminded repeatedly, or helped in doing the work itself. Stan, however, would check to see that the homework was done when he returned home in the evenings.

d. Misbehavior would not be tolerated. Anger toward a teacher or a situation would be discussed with the counselor, who would mediate when differences between the students and teachers occurred.

e. The counselor would talk with the teachers, explain the nature of the academic difficulties, and encourage them to report to the counselor when behavior improved. The counselor would then call each parent to report on the progress made.

f. In case any difficulty arose, the father as well as the mother would be informed. If possible, the father should come in to the school to deal with special situations.

g. The guidance counselor and the private therapist would

maintain weekly contact by telephone for approximately
a month and thereafter as needed. The therapist would
be informed about any group conferences concerning
the children, such as those held by the building study
team. The family and the therapist together would decide whether attendance at such meetings was to take
place.

Following the two conferences, the therapist met briefly
with just the parents for further discussion of the data. While
the information was still fresh to all, the therapist asked the
parents for their thoughts about the test results. Stan expressed the belief that the boys must have inherited his learning problems as he, too, had had such learning problems as
a boy. Laura offered the interpretation that the boys had
had little exposure to manual manipulative activity and that
the family is good at using language, especially against one
another.

When the issue of the boys' difficulties in organization was
pointed out, both parents looked at each other, recognizing
that the home is rather disorganized. Laura indicated that
she acted mostly as a troubleshooter and did not have the time
to plan ahead or to help her children be better organized.

The therapist also explained that Jeff's school was not actively involved because the school did not indicate the existence of special problems at this time. His problems, as they
were manifested at home, would be addressed during family
sessions.

G. Therapeutic Intervention with the Family

Following the school conference in which the school-based
evaluation was discussed, the family, including Jeff, attended
a session with the private therapist. The purpose of this meeting was to use the school-based data along with the therapist's
input and the family's perceptions to specify therapeutic goals.
Although the participation of all members of the family was

sought in articulating immediate goals, the therapist set out tentative short-range as well as long-range goals for change. These included the following:

a. Short-range goals

1. Work collaboratively with the school to reduce symptomatic behavior and increase productivity. This is to be enhanced by all supportive services mentioned earlier.
2. Work with the family to change the balance of involvement between the parents. Father was to take a more active role, while Mother reduced her involvement.
3. Work together with the whole family on problem-solving skills regarding homework responsibility and television scheduling.
4. Help the family plan activities that would increase their sense of cohesiveness (trips, sports, etc.).
5. Help the family develop communication skills that would enable neutral and mutual discussion of issues to replace angry outbursts.

b. Long-range goals

For the family to change it is necessary to address fundamental structural and relationship patterns. These include:

1. Work with the marital relationship by helping Stan and Laura establish clearer boundaries with their families of origin. Stan needed to invest more energy in his relationship with his nuclear family and less with his family of origin, while Laura could be helped by reconnecting with her own family of origin.
2. Stan and Laura needed to take another look at their parental roles and develop a different division of labor regarding the children.
3. Stan and Laura needed to explore their anger and critical behavior toward each other and discover its relation-

ship to their families of origin as well as alternative ways
of dealing with it.
4. Stan and Laura needed to explore the dynamics behind
   Stan's distancing posture and Laura's excessive involvement with the children. Furthermore, they needed to
   understand how their interaction reinforces each other's
   pattern of behavior.
5. The parents needed to take a look at the role played by
   each child in the totality of the family structure (e.g.,
   Jeff's acting as a third parent to his own detriment and
   to the detriment of others; and Alex and Ben taking
   turns at "highlighting" the problems in the family).

The therapist decided to structure the treatment plan along
a dual track. Weekly sessions would be held with the whole
family attending one week and the couple alone attending
on the alternate week. The focus of the family sessions would
be on the short-range issues, while the couple's sessions would
deal more extensively with the long-range goals.

Keeping these goals in mind, the therapist proceeded with
establishing communication with the family around the perception of their needs. The next few sessions were thus primarily content related and dealt with specific issues
concerning homework responsibility, television-watching,
name-calling, and bickering among the siblings. The therapist simultaneously worked on communication and problem-
solving skills. Intervention also took place to encourage Jeff
to withhold his parental role, to help Alex verbalize his angry feelings, and to help Ben hold his own so that he did not
get lost in the shuffle.

Sessions with Laura and Stan focused on practical issues of
parenting but primarily on finding ways to include Stan in
parenting activities. Thus, he took it upon himself to become the contact person with the school and to do his best
to come to the school when parental involvement was required. Laura, on the other hand, began to explore the possibility of returning to teaching on a part-time basis. The
couple also focused on issues of organization of time and
space, namely, how to maintain better physical order and

more structured activities, involving everyone in the family in determining and living up to such arrangements.

The family worked in this manner for approximately 6 months. The boys' sessions were gradually stopped, as their behavior and the quality of their work improved. Stan's involvement with his sons increased and the bond between them strengthened. Alex, in particular, developed a closer friendship with his father. (When the guidance counselor indicated to Alex that she was about ready to call his mother to tell her about his teachers' positive reports on him, he asked her to call his father instead.) The couple continued to attend therapy sessions on a biweekly basis and, at times, came in for individual sessions. The marriage was still stormy, but the couple's cooperation as parents had improved. Each was struggling to find his or her own personal power, to feel adequate as individuals, and to feel connected to each other as a family.

REFLECTIONS ON THE CASE OF THE GORDON FAMILY

It is not unusual for families to have several siblings exhibiting problems in school. From a family systems perspective, it would be rather unusual for such a phenomenon not to occur. It is also not unusual for the sibling who is functioning well at school to carry the burden of being the "normal" child. Under the surface of normalcy and productivity, one can often find a child who may be sacrificing too much of his or her own needs for the sake of the family's well-being. It is, therefore, advisable for a therapist to look into the functioning of other siblings when a referral concerning one child in the family occurs. This procedure is common practice among therapists who maintain a family systems perspective. It is less common practice, however, for the private therapist to explore the school behavior and functioning of siblings referred for private therapy.

This case illustrates the process of enlarging the therapeutic circle by taking a broad look at the total family both at home and at school.

Therapy with the Gordon family was a time-consuming intervention. However, the compensations seem to outweigh the investment. The therapist worked out of a broader spectrum of information, and the resources of the school were utilized in a coordinated manner with the therapist's work. Each party participating in the process gained optimism and courage to change because they were active participants in the process.

School personnel and therapists are not usually trained in the art of collaboration. This therapist, however, found that when given an opportunity, school personnel are most helpful and cooperative. Both therapist and school personnel can break away from the sense of isolation and find support in each other's involvement. This particular case has been an excellent learning experience for the therapist, the educators involved, and the family.

The next chapter presents a case from the point of view of the collaborative process and the central role of school personnel in initiating and carrying out the collaboration.

CHAPTER 9

CASE STUDY: OVERCOMING ABANDONMENT AND CULTURE SHOCK

with

*Julia C. Greene, C.S.W.**

The following case represents an almost idyllic collaboration experience that we would all wish for. Virtually all of the participants from the many institutions were highly competent, experienced, committed, involved, and fully cooperative in working together with an able and concerned, poor, single-parent, immigrant, multiproblem family. However, this case is not particularly exceptional within the community and organizations involved. It therefore well demonstrates the

---

* Julia C. Greene, C.S.W., is employed by the New York City Board of Education as a School Social Worker and is also a Court Evaluator and Guardian for the Association of the Bar of The City of New York. She is a noted public speaker, workshop leader, and psychotherapist/ hypnotherapist with a private practice in Queens, New York.

validity and effectiveness of the collaborative process. The collaboration in this case went on for 3½ months with a follow-up 4 months later.

BACKGROUND

A 33-year-old West Indian single mother (Mary) from a poor, overwhelmed, extended Jamaican family decided to make a better life for herself and her child (John). She took the initiative and procured a sponsor to bring her to the United States to work as a home health aid. The sponsor abandoned her shortly after her arrival. Without knowledge of how to negotiate the social system to find new employment and housing, she fell into desperate straits. Her efforts to obtain food and assistance were unsuccessful. As the pressures built up, Mary suffered a nervous breakdown and was hospitalized. Her eight-year-old son John was placed in emergency foster care.

John, too, was upset. He had been uprooted from his home and taken to an unfamiliar environment and culture where he suffered physical deprivation and watched his mother totally decompensate. He suffered the additional trauma of being separated from his mother and being placed in emergency foster care. He acted out very aggressively in school. Because of his behavioral difficulties, within one month he was placed in three different foster care settings.

After a month Mary was released from the hospital and given welfare assistance and housing. Child Protective Services now had the task of determining what to do with the child and whether the mother was capable of handling him. The social case worker for Child Protective Services/Child Welfare Association (CWA) interviewed and briefly worked with mother and child. John was tentatively returned to his mother and enrolled in a public elementary school in School District #29 in New York City in March, the last quarter of the school year. His new teacher was concerned about the boy and called the mother to discuss his fighting, other acting out behavior, and academic performance. Mary, in turn, reported the boy's problems to the CWA worker, who telephoned the school and was referred to the school social worker. Thus began a productive collaborative process.

THE PROBLEM

Of course, each participant defined the problems differently. The welfare office was interested in getting the mother sufficiently well so that she could end mental health treatment, stay out of the hospital, and get a job to support herself and her son, thereby leaving the welfare rolls. Child Protective Services was concerned about the welfare of the child. Was the mother capable of caring for him or did he need further foster-care placement? From a preventive point of view and for financial reasons, could the mother be helped to effectively care for the child? The school was interested in helping the child control his acting-out and aggressive behavior, concentrate on his work, and succeed academically.

The mother felt abandoned. She needed to know that she was not alone and that there were people who cared and would help her and her son adjust to this new culture and achieve the better life they were seeking. Mary particularly felt terribly guilty that she had failed her son. John was feeling very angry and frightened that he could lose his mother and all else that was familiar and comforting to him. He wanted a lot of reassurance that he would not be separated from his mother again and some revenge for what happened to him. He needed to control his anger and anxiety and find ways to belong in this new world. Both mother and son needed to connect with each other constructively as well as join individually with peers to overcome their isolation.

Fortunately, these disparate problems and goals were easy to mesh together in working collaboratively with this family because all parties agreed that the efforts of each reinforced the possibility of accomplishing the goals of all.

ASSESSMENT

The hospital did a full psychiatric workup on the mother during her one-month stay and with signed consent shared the findings with all concerned helpers. Mary left the hospital heavily medicated to help her control her depression and anxiety while she was assisted in making a fresh start.

The CWA worker began to see mother and child and assessed their behavior by observing them in these sessions. With informed signed consent, he too shared the information with all concerned helpers.

Since John was a new student, the current school only had information about the boy and family based upon observations and reports by the teacher and the school social worker. This information was also shared with all concerned helpers after written informed consent was obtained. Other than attendance records, little information about previous schooling was available. However, the previous school, during foster-care placement, indicated that the boy had been acting out and was being considered for special education evaluation, testing, and possible placement—a very expensive process.

Individual and family histories were obtained from the mother in interviews. The question of whether it would be wise for the family to return to their former home in Jamaica was decided in the negative because the father of the child disclaimed any responsibility for or interest in either John or Mary, and Mary's father said he could not help her.

DIAGNOSIS

The school social worker and CWA worker held telephone conferences and each met with parent and child. In these round robin meetings they all agreed that Mary's breakdown was precipitated by the social and physical stressors she experienced and that she was an intelligent, highly motivated woman who would work hard to succeed; that she needed to acquire some social supports and parenting skills; that she needed to overcome her guilt about failing her son; and that she could restore her natural self-confidence that had enabled her to have the courage to leave home and family and come with her young son to the United States.

The group further agreed that John was also intelligent and probably did not require a special education placement; that he would, however, require some help to make up his academic deficiencies; that he was suffering from the trauma of forced separation from his mother and a child's version of Post-Traumatic Stress Disorder accompanied by a great deal of anger and anxiety; that he lacked social skills and the ability to control himself in the more restrained environment of school compared with the freedom to play in Jamaica prior to starting school; that due to so many changes geographically as well as in foster-care placements, he needed stability and reassurance about his mother and other adults; and that he required structure to help him control his anxiety, anger, and behavior. Finally, all agreed that the boy had to work through his experiences and learn to trust his mother again, but that she could not avoid setting appropriate limits for him out of guilt.

TREATMENT PLAN

The plan, as described below, provided concrete services for survival and maintenance, support services to overcome isolation and improve socialization, and psychotherapy to deal with the emotional traumas. The idea was to launch an intensive all-out preventive effort to bring about rapid change based on the strengths of mother and child. Each participant agreed to carry out specific parts of the plan and to coordinate and integrate their efforts with each other, thereby reinforcing the efforts of all.

Specific aspects of the plan agreed upon involved individual therapy in a private agency and parent education in a community program for the mother; family counseling for the mother and the child in the school and a private agency; regular school placement for the child supplemented with special help from his teacher, remedial help in an At Risk Resource Room Program, and individual as well as group counseling with the school social worker; placement of the child in an after-school community tutoring and socialization program; and individual psychotherapy for the boy in a private agency.

1. Role of the Welfare Office

The Welfare Office of the New York City Department of Social Services agreed to provide a financial stipend, to obtain placement in housing, and to arrange for medical insurance through Medicaid to pay for the recommended therapy program. It followed through on all of the above and will eventually arrange and pay for additional vocational training for the mother and help her find employment.

2. Role of the School

The school social worker met with John both individually and with his mother to help them work out the separation anxiety problem that they each felt so strongly and to help the boy to adjust to his new school situation. Mary agreed to walk her son to and from school each day to reassure him, which she did. Mother and social worker engaged on setting appropriate limits for John's behavior, which the social worker also modeled during their family sessions.

The school social worker organized the school treatment plan. The teacher was informed of the problem, its origins and the joint efforts being made to help the child. She agreed to participate in the plan by being patient with John and to keep him seated very close to her so that she could more easily head off his outbursts. She further agreed to reinforce any positive behavior he manifested, while paying little attention to his less desirable behavior. The teacher carried out her part of the plan very well.

The school social worker presented the case at the Pupil Personnel Team meeting and received helpful advice and support from the team. The team agreed to place John in the At Risk Resource Room with a mature, nurturing male teacher three periods per week to learn basic skills. It was believed that once he saw he could do the work, his sense of personal competence would be reinforced. Math and reading on computer, which John loved to do, were part of the Resource Room program. It was agreed to keep him out of as many unstructured or lightly supervised situations as possible. For example, he would bring his lunch to the Resource Room rather than eat in the school cafeteria until he developed more controls. The school staff also contributed clothing for mother and son to supplement the meager social welfare benefits and to convey to the family that people cared about them.

3. Role of Community Organizations

The school social worker reached out to several community organizations to assist this family. She arranged for Mary to obtain additional needed food from a program at a local church. She further obtained admission for the boy to an afternoon tutoring and socialization program. This program was filled, but the school principal was enlisted to intervene. He succeeded in getting the boy enrolled. Here John was helped with homework and participated with other children in play and projects, giving him a chance to expend some of his considerable energy while learning to be with other children in a more informal but supervised setting.

The school social worker contacted a local community clinic and enabled Mary to attend a 10-session course in parent education. There she gained parenting skills and confidence and had an opportunity to befriend some peers. She saw that she was not alone in her situation with her son or in the community. She was extremely proud of the diploma she received on completion of the course and felt that she had truly succeeded at something important.

Finally, all participants agreed that it would be good for John to attend a summer day camp, which, after 3 months of this intensive plan, he really wanted to do. It was believed that such an opportunity would reinforce his already improving socialization skills and his self-confidence. The school social worker again stepped in and managed to get him into a local summer day camp, a funded organization in which camp tuition is free.

4. Role of Child Protective Services of the Child Welfare Administration

The CWA social worker consulted regularly with the school social worker to reassess the plan and its implementation. He accepted the agreement that the child be placed with the mother rather than in foster care. He arranged for the mother and the child to receive individual and family therapy to be paid for out of public funds. And he approved the transfer to another agency when the initial therapy agency refused to go along with the plan of seeing the mother and the child together in family therapy as part of the treatment.

5. Role of the Family

Mother and child were both active in the decision-making and problem-solving processes. They initiated ideas and proposals, evaluated the suggestions of the others, and agreed to each aspect of the treatment plan before it was implemented. Educational techniques were employed to empower the family and to emphasize their importance in the collaboration. For example, with permission the social worker modeled constructive behaviors and appropriate communication skills role-playing in session. In session, Mary and John tried out those they thought would befit them, analyzed them, and committed to practicing at home those they liked and thought would work.

Mary utilized information about nutrition: for example, that reducing John's intake of sugar could reduce his activity level and hyperactivity. It did. Mary learned to stretch her meager income by shopping with coupons available in the mail and in newspapers and by looking for items on sale. She and John clipped coupons together and felt considerable pride in their savings. Mary even used coupons from Burger King and McDonalds as part of the reward system that she developed with John for good behavior.

Mother and son together developed a reward and consequences system with very short-term objectives and goals. John realized that he could get greater attention and rewards from positive than from negative behavior.

The family initiated the idea that it would be good for John to attend a full-time summer day camp. Mary's self-esteem increased noticeably when she succeeded in getting John enrolled in a fine tuition-free camp, which involved a great deal of time, effort, and persistence on her part. After 2 months of the treatment plan, she had learned to assert herself appropriately, at least in some instances. John was happy to go to the camp, providing that his mother offered the reassurance of walking him to and from camp each day. It was a long walk and they couldn't afford a bus. Mother did accompany him. This enhanced their connection and security.

Mary was highly motivated and faithful in keeping all appointments. She carried out all agreed-upon recommendations, complied with her medication schedule, and practiced her newly acquired parenting skills. Mary supervised John's homework, set and maintained limits for him, and reconnected with him emotionally.

John took more responsibility for controlling his behavior and his anxiety. He agreed to participate in all remedial, socialization, and therapy programs and did so with a positive attitude. He accepted responsibility for his school work and his homework.

6. Role of the Therapists

All the therapists agreed to incorporate the following agenda in working with the mother: Help her to work through her own trauma and sense of abandonment, isolation, and helplessness. Relieve her of her guilt as a failure in obtaining a better life for her son. Reaffirm her intelligence and provide a lot of encouragement and positive reinforcement. Assist her to deal with and successfully negotiate the many systems in her new world. Help her identify concrete child-rearing methods that she can use, such as helping John with homework, walking him to and from school and setting appropriate limits, which, in turn, would enhance her general sense of competence and control. Improve her self-confidence, sense of competence, and general self-esteem. Help Mary reconnect appropriately with her son so that they might overcome the wounds and anxieties of the separation they had endured.

Several of the above items were to be dealt with in the mother-child sessions. The family sessions were also to focus on reinforcing their sense of family and personal stability; on classroom behavior; on how John might properly get attention from his mother and both control and release his feelings in school and at home appropriately; on immediate reinforcement of positive behavior and observance of limits set; on helping the mother verbalize her need and wishes with the boy so that she can be heard; and on labeling the son a good person who truly wants to be a good boy and make friendships with other people.

Individual therapy with the child and school social worker was to work on many of the same issues while validating the boy's trauma and helping him to express his fear and outrage about what actually happened to him. Focusing on his intelligence, the therapists could also demonstrate to him that he has now more power and control than previously because he is better able to let teachers, mother, peers, and therapists know his needs and wants.

7. Process of Coordination

The school social worker and CWA social worker took primary responsibility for coordinating the case. They held one or more weekly telephone conferences during the early assessment phase and while developing the treatment plan with the mother and child. Telephone contacts then occurred twice monthly and then ceased after a total of 4 months. The CWA counselor and school social worker each checked with the private agency therapists approximately once a month via telephone conferences.

Mother reported her activities in therapy and in the various community agencies during her regular meetings with the CWA social worker, the school social worker, and her agency therapist. The school social worker coordinated all activities with the community agencies via telephone contacts and reports from the mother. She also coordinated all activities in the school, mostly face to face with school staff members.

The school social worker conducted a follow-up of the case 4 months after her termination of it. She contacted the CWA, the psychotherapy agency, the mother, the son, and the teacher. After a discussion of some of the issues in this collaborative casework, the outcomes of the case are reported below under "Outcomes."

ISSUES

1. Conflicts

Because of the general cooperative spirit among the participants, only two conflicts arose. The most important was the refusal of the initial therapy agency to conduct family therapy sessions, which was their policy. When the others realized that part of the plan would not be implemented by this agency, the group agreed to transfer the case to another agency that specialized in dealing with families suffering neglect and deprivation and included individual and family counseling as well as parent education in their programs. It was deemed to be a better placement for the family. The second conflict occurred when the after-school program rejected the son because all of their slots were filled. Fortunately, the principal was able to prevail upon them to take one more person.

2. Different Institutional Missions

As discussed in the section on Assessment, each participating organization had different goals according to its mission

and different ways of achieving them. The family and workers were able to devise a plan that conformed to the needs of
all concerned in spite of their diversity. Each took responsibility for that part of the plan most consistent with the
organization's mission and goals. Good coordination and
follow-through also permitted each institution to reinforce
progress in ways that contributed to the progress to be
achieved by all. Thus, the family was not driven crazy by competing assertions of different pushes, pulls, and demands on
the family from each institution. Because everyone worked together, there were no opposing loyalties or demands of any kind
on anyone.

3. Record Keeping

Each organization followed its own policies in keeping
records on the case. The records, per se, were not exchanged,
although information was often and freely exchanged.

4. Ethics and Law

Child Protective Services assumed the role of insuring that
the laws pertaining to the best interests of the child were properly observed and that reasonable actions were taken to pre-
serve the family constructively intact. All parties observed
the same general ethical principles even though several different professions were involved in the case. For example,
all sharing of information was based on written informed
consent and no dual relationships were established.

OUTCOMES

1. Professional Involvement

Seven and one-half months after inception of the collaborative case, individual and family therapy at the agency were

still ongoing. Mother remained on a lower dose of medication supervised by the agency psychiatrist. The school social worker terminated the case at the end of the school year after 3½ months. The CWA worker terminated the case during the summer, satisfied that the mother was taking adequate care of her son. The after-school socialization program was terminated at the end of the school year after 3 months, but the child continued to receive help with his homework at the after-school center when the new school term began. Summer camp was terminated at the conclusion of the summer. Welfare subsidies were still being continued. The case was now being coordinated by the private agency psychotherapist basically working alone, but reporting to Medicaid and the Department of Social Services to continue with the treatment.

2. Results

John achieved well enough academically to avoid special education evaluation and placement. He was promoted to his regular grade in a regular class. His current teacher reported that he was doing satisfactory academic work but had had a few "blow-ups." However, he was in no way one of her current "problem children." Mother and child were getting along reasonably well, had no complaints, and did not feel the need for any additional help beyond Mary's individual therapy. Mother and son formed a more trusting relationship with less fear of separation from one another.

John made many friends and was very comfortable socially in his neighborhood and school. He felt connected. Mary made only one good friend who was from her parent education class. She was still vulnerable to stress and dealing with her separation/abandonment fears in therapy. Finances obviously remain tight on welfare subsidies, but the anxiety had been much reduced. Mary was looking forward to being able to go out and get a job but believed that for now she must concentrate on child rearing and making a stable home for her son. The private agency therapist agreed with this. The presenting problems have been greatly alleviated, and the plan appears to have been successful.

COST-EFFECTIVENESS

The intense short-term treatment plan has created a number of significant savings. Mother is recovering nicely and is more in control. It is unlikely that she will require further expensive hospitalization. Her improvement has made it unnecessary to place her son in foster care, which costs far more than welfare subsidies. Nor did the son require the services of testing and evaluation for special education placement or such placement itself, which are very costly to the school system.

Successful preventive therapy with the child *now* will likely head off more serious and expensive difficulties *later*. The improvement in John's school performance made it unnecessary to hold him over in the same grade the following school year, as predicted by his former school, saving the cost of an additional year of schooling. None of this includes the savings in human and institutional costs when peoples's lives and institutional activities are severely disrupted.

EVALUATION OF THE COLLABORATIVE PROCESS

It seems evident that collaboration in this case helped to achieve good results in a brief period of time with a multi-problem family in an acute crisis. It was also very cost-effective in accomplishing its multiple goals. Of course not every case is successful. In many cases the family may offer a great deal of resistance. Not every professional is equally competent or equally cooperative. Some truly prefer to be loners and to keep the total control in their own hands. Most workers are very busy and it may require a great deal of persistence to maintain their participation and active involvement.

The family in this case felt very supported by the process, and the workers reported that they, too, valued having the support of so many other resources to get the job done. Everyone could shoulder the burden, share the frustrations, and share the joy of the progress made. The process itself was felt to be enjoyable. For the agencies contracted to share the work of psychotherapy and family therapy, it was a financially profitable collaboration.

OPPORTUNITIES FOR THE PRIVATE PRACTITIONER

The school social worker indicates that in her experience most public agencies, especially in poorer neighborhoods, are overwhelmed and look for sources for referral to work with them. The school is called and the counselors, social workers, and psychologists are asked what therapists and resources are available in their community. Of course those professionals whose work is known to the school personnel are most likely to be nominated as available. Therapists who work with the school are also the most likely to be listed for referral to parents who are in need of psychotherapeutic or family therapy services. School districts typically maintain a directory of available resources. Being listed in that directory is another way to become involved in collaborative team work. Collaboration is a practice builder. Team members are constantly interreferring and enjoy working together.

CHAPTER 10

COLLEAGUES OR
COMPETITORS:
A DESIGN FOR
THE FUTURE

As our society continues to be racked by a multitude of social and economic problems, more and more children and families find themselves at risk and in distress. The preceding chapters demonstrate a rich diversity of efforts in progress by professionals of many disciplines and theoretical persuasions in different settings to reach out and meet the needs of such children and families. The underlying theme is the willingness to move beyond the closed confines of one's office and to enrich the work by collaborating with as many interested, participating parties as possible or as is effectively useful. There is also a growing recognition that one person can't do it all.

There are a number of trends that act to facilitate or to inhibit the process of cooperative problem solving to help children.

A. TRENDS THAT MAY FACILITATE
COLLABORATIVE EFFORTS

1. Moving Toward Integration of Theory and Practice Across Disciplines

Chapter 1 provides a discussion of the considerable literature on efforts toward developing integrative psychotherapy
theories, models, and modalities. The efforts of many kinds
of professionals to cross disciplinary lines to work together
as equals is cited. There is also increasing recognition that
individual, group, family, ecosystem, and psychoeducational
work all have relevance.

a. Expansion, Differentiation, and Specialization

We have experienced a century of highly creative activity
and theory building in psychotherapy with an ever-expand-
ing base of knowledge and practice skills conducted by a growing number of identified professions. We have defined many
different mental disorders or dysfunctions and labeled more
and more populations who are in need of special help. When
any field or organization gets to be too large, a typical process occurs. Increasing size produces increasing differentiation of parts within the whole, which makes it necessary to
rationalize each of the different parts and then create specialists for each of those parts.

The whole tends to get lost in a myriad of smaller parts
that are also increasing in size and further subdividing, demanding even more refined specialization and specialists.
We see this in the multiplying special interest divisions of our
major national professional organizations in mental health.
For example, the American Psychological Association now
has approximately 50 special interest divisions. We seek specialists for drug therapy, vocational counseling, abuse counseling, geriatric counseling, divorce mediation, medical social
work, child psychiatry, and neuropsychology, among a host

of others. The risk is that people become so specialized that they lose touch with the original whole and the larger wholes of which that was a part. This process inhibits collaboration.

By definition, specialization separates people and parts from the whole; it narrows down. The advantage is that specialization deepens knowledge and skills within the narrower area. Therefore, each specialist working separately may only be able to attend to one aspect of the problems represented by the child at risk. Bringing specialists together to work collaboratively means bringing together people who have more refined skills to apply cooperatively to the problem at hand. In this way, we can combine the best of all worlds.

b. Strategies to Recover the Whole

The next step is to develop strategies to recover the whole. Among the strategies used are core courses in university training programs, the acquisition of two or more disciplines by each professional, the development of hyphenated disciplines such as social psychology and behavioral medicine, and by formulating new integrative theories.

But, perhaps, what would be most helpful would be the development of new orders of generalizations cutting across theories and fields that can serve as unifying principles. For example, human behavior is clearly influenced by past history and the meanings derived from it, the present situation to be mastered, and anticipation of the future. The therapist could choose to emphasize psychogenetics, the here and now, or the process of becoming, as indeed different theories do. But is it possible that there are developmental themes such as separation and connection, with each separation opening the door to new connections, that run through the entire life cycle, around which we can organize the dimension of time? Similarly, are we not constantly faced with the struggle between stasis and change? Can we see the continuity among the constructs of self-esteem, the need to belong and feel significant in a social context, family pride, and group pride? The need for the future is such theory building.

c. Commonalities in Philosophy, Values, and Ethics

Among the helping professions there is already a commonality of philosophy evident in the large overlap to be found in the various professional codes of ethics. As a group we are people who care about others and want to do something to make lives better in this world, and we possess a strong social conscience. In turn we hold many of the same things in common with members of self-help groups. Working together with other professions can be extended to working together with self-help groups and mental health advocacy groups. The latter will have to learn to work together to share the limited resources available.

d. Identification with More Than One Profession

Another integrating factor is that many of us in mental healt h are already identified with more than one profession. The authors of this book are an example. Sherman is a licensed counseling psychologist, professor/counselor educator, family therapist, school counselor, school teacher, psychoanalyst, administrator, supervisor, author/lecturer, and private clinician. Shumsky is a licensed or certified clinical psychologist, school psychologist, family therapist, school administrator, supervisor, professor/counselor educator, author of children's literature, lecturer, and private clinician. Rountree is a licensed clinical psychologist, supervisor, professor/counselor educator, author, lecturer, and private practitioner. This crossing of boundaries makes communication and mutual interest with other professionals much easier.

2. Maintaining Equality Among Participants

The idea of a team of specialists has long been with us in hospitals, agencies, and schools. However, the team members have not generally been equal in rank. The hierarchy usually has been based upon discipline or academic degree. Parents and children have not often been invited as members of the team, and even less frequently as equal members. A major shift in thinking is required to incorporate such equality. Most of the projects described in preceding chapters do provide for collaboration among equals, including the client or patient.

3. Emphasizing Wellness and Competency

Usually, those suffering distress and dysfunction feel hurt and discouraged. Typically, the solutions already tried are not working and the participants feel stuck. They need to experience encouragement by identifying their own strengths and competencies and by being involved as competent equals in the problem-solving process. See Sherman, Oresky, and Rountree, Chapter 2 (1991) for a discussion and description of encouragement techniques. White and Epston (1990) are among the many who describe competency models of therapy. Declarations of helplessness can be countered by such methods as eliciting past successes, raising alternatives for consideration, and discussing and setting goals. The main point here is to establish some feeling of confidence and competence based upon the fact that all the people involved have some skills, strengths, and resources and, therefore, reasonable hope that the problems can be resolved. Framing issues in terms of wellness, development, prevention, and solving normal problems of the human condition is more encouraging than thinking about treatment and cure.

4. Setting Reasonable Goals for the Collaborative Work

Unfortunately, some people are beset by a host of serious problems and circumstances in their lives that would stagger almost anyone. These include multiple illnesses, deaths in the family, severe poverty, homelessness, serious addictions, physical and sexual abuse, and many others. It is not likely that the models advocated in this book are capable of coping with all the ills of society or even of a given family or child. It is important that the participants assess the situation together and determine which goals are attainable in this collaborative context. The therapist may, of course, pursue additional goals in individual or family therapy or use the models to seek collaboration with other institutions such as the courts, welfare system, hospitals, and community agencies to set and accomplish still further goals.

Goals are best described in concrete operational terms and stated in the positive rather than the negative, emphasizing what is to be done rather than what is not to be done. It is better in a first meeting to set limited and prescribed goals that are likely to succeed than to overreach and fail. If the first meeting is successful, more can be accomplished in any subsequent meeting, and the members will feel optimistic about continuing. Principles developed in the many theories of brief therapy and brief family therapy will be helpful in the setting of appropriate goals.

5. Giving More Attention to Developmental and Preventative Projects

Much of the current work is focused on crisis intervention. The pressures for this are obvious. However, it requires fewer resources to help children and families to negotiate the challenges and changes of the life cycle than to ameliorate severe dysfunction. There are many programs available that might lend themselves to collaborative projects with schools, families, couples, children, or groups of children and parents, or groups of families, or any combination of the foregoing. There are scores of commercially prepared parent education programs, couple enrichment programs, programs for children, and others for adolescents. There are programs available to address child rearing, self-esteem, divorce, grief, depression, and suicide. These commercial programs are generally well conceived and well designed. There are also many published psychoeducational programs and exercises that can be incorporated into or adapted as part of the school curriculum or as school guidance projects. Clients can be enrolled in any of the above types of programs as an adjunct to the therapy.

Freeman and Pennekamp (1988, Appendix) reproduce a chart describing preventative programs led by social workers collaborating with schools and community agencies. Among them are a project to help children who will be home alone after school, another to reduce teenage pregnancy, and a third to increase drug awareness. Freeman and Pennekamp further believe that such therapist, school, and agency coalitions in time can lead to political action to improve community conditions.

Weiss and others (1991) of the Ackerman Institute for family therapy have initiated an ambitious consultation model program in over 100 schools in the New York metropolitan area. They suggest many ways of involving parents and children in school and community projects and in school curriculum so that a community spirit is developed, which is very productive in both development and healing.

This model is described in Chapter 3. Similarly, the model developed by Comer, described in Chapter 3, seeks to organize the school and community developmentally to improve student skills, parent involvement in education, and school/community participation in the well-being of their children.

6. Caring, Hope, and Curiosity

Possibly, the most powerful motivator toward experimenting with new modalities, such as collaborative therapy with children and families at risk, is that people who enter education and therapy really want to help and succeed in helping. They care about their clients and students. They enter these professions with feelings of hope and optimism that somehow they can make a difference. Parents almost invariably want something better for their children. They hope that things will get better.

The authors believe that there are many among our colleagues who are curious to learn about new developments and to create new developments. You, the reader, are one of them or you wouldn't be bothering to read this book. Many of our colleagues are also eager to advance themselves in new ways. The modalities described herein provide for just such opportunities.

B. TRENDS THAT INHIBIT COLLABORATION

1. Protection of Turf

a. Maintaining and Enhancing the Existing Organization

A cardinal principle of systems theory is that every system or organization works to maintain itself. Maintaining itself involves establishing and protecting its identity, defining boundaries and criteria for inclusion and exclusion, providing for its economic well-being and social significance, and using strategies for its continuity. Specialized language, customs, myths, and reified ideas help to distinguish this system or organization from all others.

Initiation rites and rules of admission are designed to increase status, prestige, economic value of belonging, and to maintain a certain exclusivity. The ability to get government sanction via licensing laws is most helpful to establish legitimacy and, hopefully, some element of defined monopolistic practice (not always possible in a diverse, competitive society). These rules apply alike to professions, agencies, schools, and families. Families sanctioned by civil or religious marriage tend to be more socially advantaged than those which are not.

We regularly observe the political action of psychiatry to prevent psychologists from performing "medical practice";

the political action of psychologists, social workers, and psychiatrists to prevent or restrict the functioning of marital therapists or counselors, or the recognition of psychoanalysis as a distinct profession. However well intentioned, based upon whatever good reasons, such political actions also have the effect of attempting to establish a hierarchical pecking order of professions in which those who can maintain themselves at the top will have greater power, prestige, and earnings than those at the bottom, who will be kept out of the more lucrative and currently attractive aspects of clinical practice. Such competitive power plays mitigate against cooperative team efforts based on equality of membership.

b. The Invading of Territories

We observe how clinical psychology, which traditionally emphasized testing, assessment, and research, has strongly entered the domain of psychotherapy, formerly occupied by psychiatrists, psychiatric nurses, and social case workers. Social case workers moved from concrete social services to psychotherapy. Psychotherapists with their roots in psychoanalysis have invaded the traditional turf of counselors focusing on brief problem-solving, situationally, life-cycle oriented issues. Social workers are being strongly urged to become more involved with vocational counseling, the previously undisputed territory of vocational counselors and counseling psychologists. Members of all mental health professions are becoming increasingly involved with family therapy. Family therapists are doing more sex counseling and family therapy relative to problems traditionally within the purview of other brands of psychotherapists. These kinds of movements obviously threaten preexisting professional territories and those who would seek to protect them.

Actually, as the pace of such invasions increases, the different, distinct professions become more and more alike and the trend turns into an integrative process as well as an intense competition.

2. Competition Versus Cooperation and Collaboration

One of the many major paradoxes of our society is the effort to build all kinds of cooperative alliances within and among government, business, school, community, and family while trumpeting the ideals and practices of unfettered competition—a market economy based on survival of the fittest. We constantly hear and read that businesses should form cooperative consortia to better compete against foreign competition, while the same enterprises are in a life and death struggle against one another. Communities must compete for everything from business relocation to government grants to such natural resources as water. But they really should cooperate in ever larger units, such as in regionalization. Of course, the ultimate regions are one world and one universe. But on the other hand, a conglomerate like AT&T must be broken up into smaller, more competitive units. And world economic cartels are evil because they stifle free competition. Schools should be decentralized and made to compete with one another to improve the quality of education, but they should internally be based on cooperative team decision-making. Then there is that wonderful principle that either we'll all pull together or we'll pull apart. The push of competition makes it difficult to obey the pull of cooperation. How do we combine our wish to be a humane and compassionate society with the forces stressing survival only of the fittest?

Paradoxes like those above are confusing. Success in negotiating any paradox is to avoid the double bind of no matter what you do you lose. The lesson of the twentieth century appears to be that unrestrained competition is destructive and cooperation alone provides insufficient stimulation. Is it possible that colleagues representing different systems can come together when there is a shared interest and truly combine to assist child and family and community? There seems to be abundant evidence that competition can be put aside for common purpose. The task, then, is to define our common purpose with children at risk so that we can effectively work together.

3. Alienation Versus Connectedness

Parallel to the paradoxes of issues of competition and co-operation are those of alienation and connectedness. Many families at risk also experience themselves as somehow apart from the mainstream and, perhaps, insignificant. They have difficulty negotiating the rules of the larger systems in order to succeed and feel little or no sense of belongingness. Often social bigotry and discrimination exacerbate feelings of alienation. Lack of training in social interest and social feeling and lack of caring for others foster narcissistic behavior and insensitivity toward others. Many children and families at risk exhibit this behavior. It is easier to aggress against those who are perceived as not like you, or worse, against you. In a competitive society, others are automatically in some way against you. If this is perceived in an exaggerated form, then the individual's philosophy of life will be based on the belief that the world, or almost everyone in it, is against me. Such a person is likely to distrust any team brought together to assist him/her. They may even be hostile or overtly aggressive in the collaborative meeting format, feeling outnumbered by enemies or potential enemies. Or they may feel powerless and therefore take a very passive stance.

If the object is to include the child and family as equal problem-solvers and decision-makers, then some work needs to be done to build a greater sense of trust and empowerment in preparation for the meeting. During the meeting, their participation will be solicited, validated, and valued. Their participation will not be overshadowed by the professionals present. Nor will they be treated in a patronizing manner. The chairperson will assume major responsibility for ensuring this outcome, which will reinforce trust and empowerment and will be therapeutic in its own right.

To some degree, the professional members may experience some of the same distrust for their fellows and feel either reticent to engage fully or try to overcome the others to establish a more powerful position. Each person invited by the therapist/coordinator needs to be assured of his/her importance, potential contribution, and the rules of the game—in relation to this issue, specifically those involving equality of status.

4. Managed Care

As the health care system of this nation evolves, more and more emphasis is being put on managed care and corporate-type structures to provide, monitor, or administer the care given. This may tend to restrict the options and flexibility of practitioners employed in larger corporate provider-type units and independent practioners bound by the rules of the managers who control payment. Hopefully such managers will seek out and encourage the most effective means of providing care with the best interests of the clients in mind. Alert continuous political action in which we as professionals serve as watchdogs over the watchdogs will contribute toward that outcome.

5. Discouraging Thoughts

Other issues such as differences in cultures and ethnicity, costs, time, confidentiality, and more were discussed in Chapter 1 as issues of management. Here it is important to note that the same issues may provoke discouragement among workers to undertake collaborative programs. The therapist may think: it's too hard; it's too complicated; it's too costly; it's too risky; I won't be in control of the situation. It is the intention of this entire book to describe how to attend to such matters effectively so that they need not be sources of discouragement. As demonstrated herein, and particularly in the case studies described in Chapters 8 and 9, the task of collaborative therapy is theoretically sound, eminently practical, achievable, and profitable.

C. THE THERAPIST OF THE FUTURE

The therapist of the future will be well trained to reach out and work together with colleagues feeling self-confident in his or her own skills and neither inferior nor superior to those of other disciplines. This therapist will respect the strengths and resources that colleagues can provide. The therapist will also be a good problem-solver and coordinator and will find that working together is stimulating, exciting, and growth producing and will firmly place him or her in a network of caring professionals with whom to share. Burn-out will be a less frequent phenomenon because of the cooperative support systems of which he or she is an active part. Participation in such networks will greatly increase the therapist's visibility, effectiveness, and reputation leading to a solid referral base to support the practice and keep it growing to the desired size.

The therapist of the future will be less stressed because of the support of her fellows, the shared responsibility for outcomes, and a collaborative process in which leadership and initiative-taking may flow naturally among the participants.

The therapist of the future will enjoy greater overall success with clients. By working collaboratively with clients as equals, all share together the responsibility for the success of the enterprise. The therapist of the future will share his or her optimism and belief that clients are worthy people who have strengths, resources, and ideas that can be elicited and brought to bear to improve themselves and their situation and that they are indeed equal partners in the search for better ways of being and doing.

In connecting as equals with a collaborative team the clients will know that they are not alone and will find that very encouraging. Those feelings of encouragement will serve as a tonic for the professionals who will also feel the same sense of connectedness and encouragement in their work. The meshing of curiosity and cooperative brainstorming will lead to new insights and patterns of behavior. The modeling that takes place in the team enterprise will be in itself a refreshing experience of good human relationships that can have vital carryover effects in the lives of all, including the personal growth of the therapist.

It could happen to you.

Bibliography

Albert, L. (1989). *A teacher's guide to cooperative discipline.* Circle Pines, MN: American Guidance Service.

Allen, D. M. (1988). *Unifying individual and family therapy.* San Francisco: Jossey-Bass.

Ansbacher, H. L., & Ansbacher, R. R. (Eds.). (1956). *The individual psychology of Alfred Adler: A systematic presentation in selections from his writings.* New York: Basic Books.

Atteneave, C. (1976). Social networks as the unit of intervention. In R. J. Guerin (Ed.), *Family therapy: Theory and practice.* New York: Gardner Press.

Beal, E. W., & Chertkov, L. S. (1992). Family-school intervention: A family systems perspective. In M. J. Fine & C. Carlson (Eds.), *The handbook of family-school intervention: A systems perspective* (pp. 288–301). Boston: Allyn and Bacon.

Boszormenyi-Nagy, I. & Spark, G. (1984). *Invisible loyalties: Reciprocity in intergenerational family therapy (2nd ed.).* New York: Brunner/Mazel.

Bowen, M. (1978). *Family therapy in clinical practice.* New York: Jason Aronson.

Boyd-Franklin, N. (1989). *Black families in therapy: A multisystems approach.* New York: Guilford Press.

Carl, D., & Jurkovic, G. J. (1983). Agency triangles: Problems in agency-family relationships. *Family Process, 22(4),* 441–451.

Carlson, D. (1992). Models and strategies of family-school assessment and intervention. In M. J. Fine & C. Carlson (Eds.), *The handbook of family-school intervention: A systems perspective* (pp. 18–44). Boston, MA: Allyn & Bacon.

Carter, B., & McGoldrick, M. (Eds.). (1988). *The changing family life cycle: A framework for family therapy (2nd ed.).* New York: Gardner Press.

Christensen, O. C. & Schramski, T. G. (1983). *Adlerian family counseling.* Minneapolis, MN: Educational Media Corp.

Comer, J. P. (1988). Educating poor minority children. *Scientific American, 259(5),* 42–48.

Comer, J. P. (1993). A brief history and summary of the School Development Program: 1992–1993. Unpublished manuscript.

Comer, J. P., & Haynes, N. M. (1992). Summary of School Development Program (SDP) effects. Unpublished manuscript.

Dinkmeyer, D., & Sherman, R. (1989). Brief Adlerian family therapy. *Individual Psychology: The Journal of Adlerian Theory, Research and Practice, 45 (1 & 2),* 148–158.

Elizur, J., & Minuchin, S. (1990). *Institutionalizing madness: Family theory and society.* New York: Basic Books.

Family Therapy News (1991, June). Special issue.

Feldman, L. B. (1991). *Integrating individual and family therapy.* New York: Brunner/Mazel.

Freeman, E. M., & Pennekamp, M. (1988). *Social work practice: Toward a child, family, community perspective.* Springfield, IL: Charles C Thomas.

Gatti, F., & Colman, C. (1988). Community network therapy: An approach to aiding families with troubled children. In W. M. Walsh & N. J. Giblin (Eds.), *Family counseling in school settings* (pp. 132–144). Springfield, IL: Charles C Thomas.

Gergen, K. J. (1991). *The saturated self: Dilemmas of identity in contemporary life.* New York: Basic Books.

Golden, L. B. (1984). Quick assessment of family functioning. *The School Counselor, 18,* 179–183.

Goldenberg, I., & Goldenberg, H. (1991). *Family therapy: An overview* (3rd ed.). Pacific Grove, CA: Brooks/Cole.

Gurman, A. S., & Kniskern, D. P. (Eds.). (1991). *Handbook of family therapy* (Vol. 2). New York: Brunner/Mazel.

Haley, J. (1976). *Problem-solving therapy: New strategies for effective family therapy.* San Francisco: Jossey-Bass.

Hartman, A. (1979). *Finding families: An ecological approach to family assessment in adoption.* Beverly Hills, CA: Sage.

Hawkins, J. L. (1993). Hanging out: An intervention for random families. In T. S. Nelson & T. S. Trepper (Eds.), *101 interventions in family therapy* (pp. 59–62). New York: Haworth Press.

Haynes, N. M., & Comer, J. P. (1990). The effects of a school development program on self-concept. *The Yale Journal of Biology and Medicine, 63,* 275–283.

Haynes, N. M., Comer, J. P., & Hamilton-Lee, M. (1989). School climate enhancement through parental involvement. *Journal of School Psychology, 8(4),* 291–299.

Hoffman, L. (1981). *Foundations of family therapy.* New York: Basic Books.

Imber-Black, E. (1988). *Families and larger systems: A family therapist's guide through the labyrinth.* New York: Guilford Press.

Kern, R. M., Hawes, E. C., & Christensen, O. C. (Eds.). (1989). *Couples therapy: An Adlerian perspective.* Minneapolis, MN: Educational Media Corp.

Koizumi, E. (1990). School nonattendance and psychological and counseling services. In C. Chiland & J. G. Young (Eds.), *Why children reject school: Views from seven countries* (pp. 88–97). New Haven, CT: Yale University Press.

Kral, R. (1986). Indirect therapy in the schools. In S. DeShazer and R. Kral (Eds.), *Indirect approaches in therapy.* Rockville, Md: Aspen Press.

Levant, R. E. (1984). *Family therapy: A comprehensive overview.* Englewood Cliffs, NJ: Prentice-Hall.

Lightfoot, S. L. (1978). *Worlds apart: Relationships between families and schools.* New York: Basic Books.

Lusterman, D-D. (1985). An ecosystemic approach to family-school problems. *American Journal of Family Therapy, 13,* 22–30.

Lusterman, D-D. (1988). School-family interaction and the circumplex model. *Journal of Psychotherapy and the Family, 4,* 267–283.

Lusterman, D-D. (1991, October). Between school and family: A place for family therapists. *Family Therapy News,* pp. 3–4.

Lusterman, D-D. (1992). Ecosystemic treatment of family-school problems: A private practice perspective. In M. J. Fine & C. Carlson (Eds.), *The handbook of family-school intervention: A systems perspective* (pp. 363–373). Boston: Allyn and Bacon.

Meyer, C. H. (Ed.). (1983). *Clinical social work in the ecosystems perspective.* New York: Columbia University Press.

Minuchin, P. (1992). A systems approach to foster care. *Prevention Report.* University of Iowa School of Social Work, National Resource Center of Family Based Services. Fall, pp. 1–3.

Minuchin, S. (1974). *Families and family therapy.* Cambridge, MA: Harvard University Press.

Minuchin, S., & Fishman, H. C. (1981). *Family therapy techniques.* Cambridge, MA: Harvard University Press.

Murase, K. (1990). School refusal and family pathology: A multifaceted approach. In C. Chiland & J. G. Young (Eds.), *Why children reject school: Views from seven countries* (pp. 73–87). New Haven, CT: Yale University Press.

Nakane, A. (1990). School refusal: Psychopathology and natural history. In C. Chiland & J. G. Young (Eds.), *Why children reject school: Views from seven countries* (pp. 62–72). New Haven, CT: Yale University Press.

Nelson, T., & Trepper, T. S. (Eds.). (1993). *101 interventions in family therapy.* New York: Haworth Press.

Nichols, M. (1987). *The self in the system: Expanding the limits of family therapy.* New York: Brunner/Mazel.

Nichols, W.C., & Deissler, K.G. (Eds.). (1988). Power and family therapy. *Journal of Contemporary Family Therapy: An International Journal, 10,* 2.

Nicoll, W. (1984). School counselors as family counselors: A rationale and training model. *The School Counselor, 18,* 279–283.

Nicoll, W. G., Platt, J. M., & Platt, A. (1983). Adlerian programs in the schools. In O. Christensen & I. Schramski (Eds.), *Adlerian family counseling: A manual* (pp. 317–342). Minneapolis, MN: Educational Media Corp.

O'Brien, C. (1976). A school counselor calls for help. *Journal of Family Counseling, 4,* 75–77.

O'Callaghan, J. B. (1993). *School-based collaboration with families: Constructing family-school-agency partnerships that work.* San Francisco, CA: Jossey Bass.

Olson, D. (1986). Circumplex model VII: Validation studies and FACES III. *Family Process, 25,* 337–351.

Pflaum, S. W., & Longo, P. (1989, January). *Shared commitments: The collaboration of I.S. 227Q and Queens College.* Unpublished manuscript, School of Education, Queens College, City University of New York.

Rueveni, D. (1979). *Networking families in crisis.* New York: Garland.

Schaeffer, C. E. (Ed.). (1988). *Innovative interventions in child and adolescent therapy.* New York: Wiley.

Scharff, D. E., & Scharff, J. S. (1987). *Object relations family therapy.* Northvale, NJ: Aronson.

Schmidt, J. J. (1993). *Counseling in schools: Essential services and comprehensive programs.* Boston: Allyn and Bacon.

Seeman, M. (1968). Alienation and social learning in a reformatory. *American Journal of Sociology, 18,* 189–196.

Sherman, R. (1983). Power in the family: An Adlerian perspective. *The American Journal of Family Therapy, 11(3),* 43–53.

Sherman, R., & Dinkmeyer, D. (1987). *Systems of family therapy: An Adlerian Integration.* New York: Brunner/Mazel.

Sherman, R., & Fredman, N. (1986). *Handbook of structured techniques in marriage and family therapy.* New York: Brunner/Mazel.

Sherman, R., Oresky, P., & Rountree, Y. (1991). *Solving problems in couples and family therapy: Techniques and tactics.* New York: Brunner/Mazel.

Silber, J. T. (1993). Innovative children's mental health policy arrives. *Family Therapy News, 24(3),* 5, 12.

Speck, R., & Atteneave, C. (1973). *Family networks.* New York: Pantheon.

Spillane, M. (Ed.). (1992). SDP launches video series. *School Development Program Newsline, 1(2),* 1–8.

Stanton, J. L., & Stanton, M. D. (1984). *Pick-a-Dali-Circus.* Workshop held at the national convention of the American Association for Marriage and Family Therapy.

Steele, W., & Raider, M. (1991). *Working with families in crisis: School-based intervention.* New York: Guilford Press.

Tagiuri, R. (1968). The concept of organizational climate. In R. Tagiuri & G. H. Litwin (Eds.), *Organizational climate: Exploration of a concept* (pp. 10–32). Cambridge, MA: Harvard University Press.

Wachtel, P. L., & Wachtel, E. F. (1986). *Family dynamics in individual therapy.* New York: Guilford.

Wang, M. C. (1992). *Comprehensive approach to schooling success project.* Unpublished abstract, Temple University Center for Research in Human Development and Education, Philadelphia.

Weiss, H. M., & Edwards, M. E. (1992). *The family-school collaboration project: Systemic interventions for school improvement.* In S. Christenson & J. C. Conoley (Eds.), *Home-school collaboration: Enhancing children's academic and social competence.* Colesville, MD: National Association for School Psychologists.

Weiss, H. M., Edwards, M. E., & Schwartz, A. (1991). Systemic interventions produce innovative school change. *Family Therapy Forum, 9–12.*

White, M., & Epston, D. (1990). *Narrative means to therapeutic ends.* New York: Norton.

Williams, G., Robinson, F., & Smaby, M. (1988). School counselors using group counseling with family-school problems. *The School Counselor, 22,* 170–177.

Woody, R. H., Yeager, M., & Woody, J. D. (1990). Appropriate education for handicapped children: Introducing family therapy to school-based decision making. *American Journal of Family Therapy, 18,* 189–196.

Appendix: Examples of Permission Forms

Request for Data from Another Therapist or Institution

Name of Therapist and/or Institution
Address
Telephone Number

CONSENT FORM FOR THE RELEASE OF INFORMATION

Date_____

I (we) hereby give informed written consent to (*Name and address of therapist or institution to GIVE the information*)

_____

_____

to release and provide all pertinent information requested pertaining to my (our) case to (*Name of person or institution SENDING FOR the information*) at the address on the letterhead above for purposes of: (*i.e. building more effectively on previous case history; better placement; better case coordination, supervision; or use in psychotherapy or family therapy.*)

_____

_____

Your cooperation is appreciated.
Thank you.

(Client Signatures)

_____

_____

In accordance with the above release:
__ I will call to arrange a telephone interview.
__ Please send a copy of the complete file.
__ Please send copies of available reports or records.
__ Please send a written report on the case.

Thank you,
Name of person requesting the data
Title _____

187

Receiving Permission from Clients to Send Data to Others

Name of Therapist or Institution
Address
Telephone Number

CONSENT FORM FOR THE RELEASE OF INFORMATION

Date_____

I (we) hereby give informed written consent to (*insert name of therapist or institution*), above address, to release and provide all pertinent information requested about me (us) and my (our) case to:

(*Insert name and address of therapist[s] or institutions to receive the information*)

_____
_____
_____

for the purpose of:

_____
_____

The purpose for which this information is being requested has been fully explained to me (us) and is fully understood.

Signed   _____

_____
_____

Name Index

Subject Index

Abuse, 61; emotional, 2; physical, xv, 2; sexual, 2; substance, xv, 2, 8, 11, 64, 78, 79, 81, 91
Accountability, 17–18, 59, 86
Ackerman Family Institute's School Collaboration Model, 49, 51–55, 67, 68
Acting-out, 35
Adaptability, 107–108
Adaptation, cultural, 2
Adlerian Consultation Model, 49, 55–58
Administrative subsystems: hierarchies in, 45; triadic interventions in, 45–46
Alcohol abuse, 11, 78
Alienation, 12, 52, 54, 71, 91, 177–178
Alliances, 30–32, 63
Anxiety, separation, 84–85
ASPECTS 27 Model, 69, 77–79
Assessment, 154; cognitive function, 104–107; collaboration in, 103–119; level of adaptability, 107–108; process, 103–119; school, 130–135; social and emotional function, 107–119
At-risk children: criteria for, xv; identification of, 91–92; referral for therapy, 96; school alienation in, 6
Attendance, 72, 77

Attention deficit, 38, 39, 104–105
Authority, 32–33, 110–111; in administrative subsystems, 45; attitudes toward, 39, 72; challenging, 111; changing structures, 83; defiance of, 91; parental, 84
Autism, 35
Autonomy, 62, 63, 108–109
Avoidance, 64

Behavior: adaptive, 107–108; addictive, 11; avoidant, 87; classroom, 72; cognitive aspects, 38; defensive, 87; dynamics of, 57; enabling of, 11; family, 71; holistic thinking about, xvi, 76, 77; human, 24; influence of organizations on, xvi; interpretation of, 83; listening, 104–105; modification, 82–83; nonconforming, 91; oppositional, 107; parental, 11; patterns, xvi, 39, 50; perceptions of, 34; purposes of, 55; rating scales, 104; rebellious, 6; reciprocal, 1, 10; reinforcing, xvi, 10, 11; repeating pattern of, 10; self-defeating, 64, 66; social context of, xv;

Milton Keynes UK
Ingram Content Group UK Ltd.
UKHW031134141024
449569UK00006B/183